THE
BODY
RESET
Diet

Power Your Metabolism, Blast Fat, and Shed Pounds in Just 15 Days

HARLEY PASTERNAK, MSc
with Laura Moser

RODALE

To my beautiful wife, Jessica, who provides me with boundless love, inspiration, laughter, and chocolate chip cookies.

Contents

PART III
THE REST OF YOUR LIFE

Acknowledgments

My literary agent, Andy Barzvi, who believed in me first, then made sure everyone else did too.

My family for keeping me grounded.

Andre Hudson. Your energy, loyalty, and laughter is invaluable.

Wendy Heller for being half lawyer and half sister.

Nancy Fowler, Holly Rawlinson, and Steve Fowler for tirelessly turning my little ideas into big businesses.

Laura Moser for helping me find the words . . . then putting them in the right order.

Susan Ott for the delicious recipes.

Ursula Cary and the team at Rodale Books for making this book become a reality.

Allison Garfield, for editing my edits.

Shelley Linden for letting me cheat off her in organic chemistry class.

The Ladies of the Revolution for inspiring me.

Tara Piper for keeping me hydrated.

Jen Hamel-Keddy for making sure I always have the coolest shoes.

Introduction

As a culture, we've gone *way* overboard trying to beat the bulge. We've spent too much money, time, and effort trying to get thin. We've gone on all sorts of diets—low cal, low carb, low fat—in the hopes of achieving our dream body. We've popped endless pills and cleansed our insides until nothing's left. We've eaten according to our blood type, subsisted on grapefruits for months on end, and come very close to starving ourselves. Why do we keep on getting fatter and fatter? Why is it that the country with the most gyms, health foods, low-cal salad dressings, and diet gurus on earth can't seem to stop gaining weight?

We all know how fat we are as a country: More than one-third of US adults, a whopping 35.7 percent, are not just overweight but *obese*, and that already-shocking figure is expected to rise to 42 percent by the year 2030.[1] But if we're so aware of the problem, why can't we seem to do anything to fix it?

Before we do anything else, we need to stop, take a step back, and look at what we're actually doing.

Let's agree that we're confused. The competing information we're being bombarded with day and night isn't doing us any good. The Internet is great for streaming my favorite shows and finding out the weather, but when it comes to disseminating the right information about health and fitness, it's nothing if not bewildering and even downright dangerous. Let's just forget what we've heard—everything we know, or thought we knew.

We need to hit the reset button.

We need to reset the way we think about food.

We need to reset our metabolism.

We need to reset our bodies.

All of us, including me. That's right: Despite having espoused a healthy, moderate lifestyle over the last 20 years, I have realized that moderation isn't always enough, at least not as the first step toward real weight loss. Ultimately, moderation *is* the key to success. But while a more gradual approach to weight loss by working out five times a week and eating five balanced meals a day is incredibly effective for long-term weight loss, I have come to understand the urgent desperation so many of you feel—YOU WANT TO LOSE WEIGHT NOW! Not next month, or even next week. Today. *This afternoon.* This conviction was deepened by a recent study that found people who lose a significant amount of weight early on in a weight-loss plan are far likelier to stick with the plan over the long run.[2]

That was certainly my experience working on the personal transformation show *The Revolution* on ABC, which was in many ways a life-changing experience for me. I saw over and over again that the women who lost the most weight right away were the ones who stuck with the program over the long haul, well after the TV show had ended. I saw, in other words, that instant gratification *works.* No, quick fixes might not be ideal, but we need to see results to stay motivated. That's just how human nature operates.

I set out to create the plan of all plans, a plan that brought immediate and dramatic results, without compromising participants' health or leading to that disastrous yo-yo effect (lose 10 pounds this week, regain

15 next week) associated with so many diets. The plan I've devised is so simple yet so effective that you will *immediately* lose weight regardless of any reasons you may have failed in the past.

I call it *The Body Reset Diet.* As you make your way through the program, you'll be shocked by how effortlessly the pounds seem to fall off. You'll also be shocked that you can build a lean, sexy body without investing in expensive equipment or waking up at 5 a.m. to do crazy things like one-handed pushups in boot camp for an hour.

Most of all, you'll be shocked that when you follow this plan, you will experience no deprivation, only gratification. You will be satisfied by how good you look and how alive you feel, and you will be motivated to keep going.

This plan is so easy that you'll forget you're even on a plan. All it takes is a few minutes of food prep, a few minutes of structured exercise, and a commitment to get out there and get walking—I promise that nothing could be simpler or more effective.

But before embarking on the Body Reset, you must *believe* that you can lose weight. That you can transform your body, that you can be stronger and more energetic. You have to believe that in just 15 days you can be on the road to the best health—and the best body—of your life.

So before we get started, repeat after me: "I CAN look and feel better."

Now, replace that "CAN" with "WILL" and say it out loud: "I WILL look and feel better!"

Do you feel a difference between the two statements?

Many weight-loss programs CAN possibly make you look and feel better for a short period of time. Your decision to follow the Body Reset Plan WILL make you look and feel better, now and forever.

I

A New Kind
of Diet

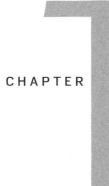

CHAPTER

Why Diets Fail

Many people tell me, *Harley, I've done every diet you can think of!* Take my word for it—in the long run, none of them work. Well, obviously they didn't work, or you wouldn't be reading this book. Or maybe they worked for a week or two before your weight boomeranged back to its usual (depressing) number on the scale, but the end result is the same: You think you're doing everything right, and you still can't lose the weight. And after a while, you become discouraged—and why wouldn't you?

Why does nothing you've tried work? You've attempted so many diets that you can no longer open your refrigerator door without feeling a massive headache clamp down. There is SO much competing information out there, and so many contradictory recommendations, that it's no wonder we no longer have any idea what we're supposed to eat or how we're supposed to move. Eat low carb. Eat no carbs. Eat ALL carbs. . . . Who could possibly make sense of all these competing prescriptions?

Did you know that more than half of Americans, an astonishing 52 percent, think it's easier to do their own income taxes than to figure out how to eat healthier? That's right, filing with the IRS has suddenly become preferable to knowing what you should have for lunch.[1]

Let me tell you: It's time to stop. Enough is enough! We are listening to the wrong people telling us to do the wrong things. Who are these authorities, anyway? A lot of the TV trainers we're letting guide our fitness decisions are straight out of central casting (and I mean literally straight out of central casting) meaning they have zero credentials in the field of nutrition and have never trained anyone in their lives before their first television appearance.

I had the privilege of hosting a talk-show called *The Revolution,* which was one of the most rewarding experiences of my professional career. The amazing women I met helped me rethink my whole weight-loss philosophy. Even with 10 years of education and 20 years in my practice, I needed to change my way of thinking. That's a lot more than I can say about most of the high-profile "experts" who are dictating the health decisions too many people are making.

It's my training, and the wide range of people whose bodies and minds I've helped transform over the past 20 years, from Halle Berry and Jessica Simpson to single-mom schoolteachers, that has led me to understand exactly how serious the crisis we're facing is. Let me tell you, I know exactly what you're going through, whether you need to lose a ton of weight, or those last stubborn 5 pounds, and you have no idea where to begin. That's what I'm here for. Stick with me for the next 15 days and you will see amazing, dramatic results—in your energy level, in your health, and most noticeably in your weight.

To get there, first we have to wipe the slate clean. Press reset. Start over. Rethink everything you've ever been told about how to lose weight. People are looking to crazier diet solutions than ever, and where is it getting them? Right back where they started from—maybe even a few pounds heavier. So before you embark on your next crazy scheme, let me explain why you keep failing, and why you can see far more dramatic results from a much simpler and more sensible approach.

Trust me, I realize what I'm up against because I know exactly how much crazy stuff is out there. I admit that some of the better-known, more mainstream programs—with point systems and so forth—can be effective, but in many cases they take too long for the kind of results people want (and deserve), and some are also prohibitively expensive.

So people turn to the more extreme quick fixes, everything from eating like a caveman to inserting feeding tubes in their arms and living off nothing but liquids in IV form for weeks on end. I mean—are you serious? Losing weight does not have to resemble an all-out death wish.

The caveman lived on nuts and meats alone, but he also stayed active all day long and—oh, yeah—he generally died by age 18! In all other ways, our lives are hardly Paleolithic: We pop countless pills in the hopes of losing a few pounds here and there. Weight-loss pills are a *$2.4 billion* industry in the United States, despite a recent study determining that no evidence exists that any single product will result in significant weight loss.[2] Even sketchier is that some bodybuilding and weight-loss pills have been shown to cause liver damage, among other serious health issues.[3]

Weight-loss pills are often unregulated and can be quite dangerous. From 1999 to 2008, the U.S. Food and Drug Administration (FDA) received 32 reports of serious liver damage in people taking orlistat, the active ingredient in Alli weight-loss pills; 27 patients were hospitalized and six cases resulted in liver failure. The FDA says it's not completely clear if orlistat caused the liver damage and is not telling people taking

Xenical or Alli to stop using the weight-loss pills. But the agency warns them to be careful to use the medicine as directed.[4] It's clear that using weight-loss pills can cause serious damage and just aren't worth the risk to your health.

What about attempting to cleanse your body of all those toxins that must surely be the sole reason for your bloat? Detox cleanses have gotten huge in recent years, propelled by promises of quick results and endorsed by top celebrities. But the days upon days of near-fasting recommended by these programs can have some seriously nasty side effects, including vitamin deficiencies, muscle breakdown, blood sugar problems, loose stool, and overall weakening of the body's immune system and ability to fight infection and inflammation. Excessive cleansing can also lead to the expulsion of "good bacteria," which are essential for keeping the intestines healthy and the whole immune system functioning properly.

When you're coping with all these issues—and I haven't even mentioned the headaches, irritability, fatigue, aches and pains, and dehydration—how are you supposed to carry on with the rest of your life, much less get the exercise you need to be healthy? And how can you *possibly* stay on any such extreme plan for more than a few agonizing days?

The answer is: You can't, and that's why you're reading this book. These quick fixes might help you squeeze back into your favorite jeans by Friday night, but they are wreaking major havoc on your health, and the results DO NOT LAST, for a whole multitude of reasons.

Here's where the yo-yo-ing comes in. You lose 15 pounds by surviving (barely) on grapefruits for a month, but then within hours of putting real food in your poor depleted body again, your weight immediately balloons up 20 pounds above your original starting point. How else is your poor confused metabolism supposed to react?

So let's give up all this crazy stuff. *None of it works.* It's just crazy.

REASONS DIETS FAIL

They Require Too Much Time, Effort, or Money

Many diets, including some of the healthier, moderation-based plans, fail because they ask too much of the participants' time. Whether it's attending meetings during lunch hour, writing down and adding up every single bite of food consumed over the course of the day, or spending an hour of prep time per recipe five times a day, many of these diets make unreasonable demands on our already-crammed schedules. I just opened up a hot new diet cookbook and the first recipe I saw was for an omelet—with 12 ingredients! (P.S. I made it, and it was gross. Thanks for nothing, firefighter diet.) However noble their aims, these diets simply ask too much of us. Most of us are already juggling enough responsibilities as it is.

Learning how to eat efficiently and move effectively is not rocket science, but we've complicated everything so much that it's sometimes hard to see the forest for the trees. When you don't succeed on a diet, it's not because you're a fundamentally weak person; it's because you've set yourself up to fail with endless impossible restrictions and headache-inducing do-and-don't lists.

The other problem with diets tends to be price. They just cost too much. Getting ready-made meals delivered to your door might be convenient, but it sure isn't cheap. A recent study examined 10 of the most popular diets and found that their median cost was $85.79 per week, or roughly 58 percent more than the average $54.44 most Americans spend weekly on food. And some—like the Jenny Craig diet, which has an average cost of $137.65 per week—are even pricier still.[5] One popular detox cleanse costs an eye-popping $195 for a 3-day supply of juice.

That's almost $70 a day—a huge financial commitment for some seriously dubious rewards.

They Teach the Wrong Lessons About Food

Whether you're eating all juice, all cereal, or all red meat, eventually your palate will rebel against the monotony. It's perfectly natural for you to get sick of eating the exact same ingredient over and over again,

The more restrictive the diet, it seems, the more likely the weight loss is temporary. According to recent research published in *American Psychologist*, while people can lose 5 to 10 percent of their weight in the first few months of a diet, up to two-thirds of them regain even more weight than they lost within 4 or 5 years.[6]

Many diets ignore the fact that eating is one of the great pleasures in life by depriving dieters of a huge range of foods, and no one can possibly stay on such a limiting regimen for so long. It doesn't help that most foods on these programs don't taste good. When you're living off space-food-like prepackaged frozen entrees or raw kale salad all day, you're not going to look forward to your meals—and why would you? You eat this way because you want to lose weight, but after the first few days the very idea of another frozen chicken dish and/or bowl of steamed bok choy and watercress makes your stomach turn, and so you stray from your plan for one meal and then another, and before the week is up you're off the program altogether.

Other diets demand we hunt down hard-to-find, exotic ingredients— as if, if your local grocery store doesn't happen to carry organic free-range venison, quail eggs, or persimmons, your whole eating plan is doomed on Day 1.

They Confuse Some Basic Nutritional Facts

Some diet programs focus exclusively on the old "calories in, calories out" rule, the theory being that if you expend more calories than you take in, you will lose weight, period, end of story. But diets that focus exclusively on calories and not what those calories are made of are completely misguided. I cannot emphasize this point enough: *Not all calories are created equal.*

Fourteen hundred calories of white bread is NOT the equivalent of fourteen hundred calories of salmon. Different foods affect our bodies differently, regardless of caloric content. They make you look different and feel different, too.

A recent study found that following a low-fat diet can slow down your metabolism, which makes weight loss more difficult, whereas a high-protein diet can increase the body's fat-burning capabilities.[7] Another found that low-fat diets are *not* the best route to lasting weight loss.[8] So losing weight is not a simple matter of caloric arithmetic. You also have to consider WHAT you're eating, not just how much of it.

And far too often, diets deprive us not only of calories but of the foods we need to live at the top of our game. If, for example, you're on a juice fast, you're not getting ANY protein, healthy fats, or fiber—and your body needs all of these nutrients to function. Because you're depriving your body, you'll probably be hungry, miserable—and extremely vulnerable to falling off the wagon. We also don't take in enough liquids, and many of us live in a state of semidehydration, which our bodies far too often confuse for hunger, which causes us to eat more.

"While struggling with my weight, I had turned to many different programs. They all left me feeling like a failure, and I was even considering surgical weight-loss options. Harley's plan saved me. It gave me the tools and knowledge I needed to find a healthy way of living. I have never felt so alive as I do today, and I know that I am a success."

—Nancy Daly, *lost 20 pounds in 15 days*

They Push Exercise Too Much

Never thought you'd hear that from a fitness professional, did you? But overexercising can be a real problem. First off, no amount of exercise can undo the effects of a bad diet. Do you know how many minutes you have to do on an elliptical trainer to offset the caloric burden of a single slice of cheesecake? Up to an hour and a half. And no studies have shown that exercise in and of itself definitively causes weight loss. As Gary Taubes put it in his well-argued book *Why We Get Fat*, "very little evidence exists to support the belief that the number of calories we expend"—i.e., how much we work out—"has any effect on how fat we are."[9]

I believe it's because our over-the-top workout habits end up supercharging our appetites, ultimately causing us to consume even more calories than we would have if we'd stayed home and skipped the gym. Taubes once again states the case plainly: "Increase the energy you expend and the evidence is very good that you will increase the calories you consume to compensate."[10] Put in the simplest terms possible: The harder you work out, the hungrier you'll be, and the more you eat. But if you want to lose weight, increasing the number of calories you're taking in is counterproductive at best.

I started thinking about this seeming contradiction more and more in the summer of 2009, when *Time* published a cover story called "Why Exercise Won't Make You Thin."[11] The gist was—hey, it's great that you go to the gym, but if you leave the gym famished and hit the all-you-can-eat buffet on your way home, you're still going to gain weight, simple as that.

But was it? Why have so many popular fitness programs failed to get this message? Turn on your TV and look at all the current exercise infomercials out there—ever tried working out with that drill sergeant shouting orders at you to do nearly impossible types of exercise at nearly impossible levels of intensity with no regard for possibility of injury? Many of these programs are way too difficult, way too intense, and there's just no method to the madness. I myself am in great shape and can't do most of these exercises! Why is there a program based on chinups when only a tiny percentage of the population can actually do these incredibly advanced exercises?

Far too often, this radical approach to exercise—the extreme boot camps, the triathlon training, the scary DVD programs that sound like cruise missiles—has another unfortunate unintended consequence. It can lead to an explosion in sports injuries, back problems, and tendinitis, which in turn impedes one's ability to maintain physical activity over the long term. Our recent (and ever-growing) passion for marathons and Iron Man competitions and other such "extreme endurance exercise" can have serious negative effects on our bodies, leading to structural changes to our heart and large arteries, as a recent study found.[12] It's no big shocker that emergency-room visits resulting from weight training rose nearly 50 percent between 1990 and 2007.[13] We are pushing ourselves too far, and for no good reason.

They Don't Make Us Exercise *Enough*

The flipside of the tendency to overexercise is that most of us don't exercise *enough*—even those of us who devotedly attend a kickass spin class after work every night. Sound like a contradiction? It's not. Regular gym attendance can in no way compensate for an otherwise completely sedentary lifestyle. And for far too many of us, sedentary is the norm. Thanks to the Internet, cell phones, and all the other technologies that rule our days, most of us can get through the workday without once getting up from our desk. We can buy our clothes and even our groceries without taking a step. These technological advances have made our workdays more efficient, but what are they doing to our bodies?

If we drive everywhere and sit at a desk all day, then return home to sit on a couch all night, we are going to gain weight. Period. It really is that simple. A recent Finnish study found that, while regular exercise is important for health, long bouts of physical inactivity can be hazardous *even if the person also exercises.*[14] And a recent study in the *Lancet* concluded that lack of exercise can be as hazardous to the health as smoking, responsible for as many as 1 in 10 premature deaths, with 5.3 million of the 57 million deaths in 2008 being attributed to conditions like heart disease and diabetes.[15]

Most diet plans fail to take into account the importance of regular movement in maintaining a healthy weight. When you are starving yourself half to death, you seldom have the energy to move, and when you fail to move, you quickly lose your lean muscle tissue, which in turn makes your resting metabolism go down, which in turn makes it harder for your body to lose weight. Seriously, try doing any sustained exercise, much less doing daily household chores, when you haven't eaten in almost 2 weeks. It's not going to happen.

Again, the Internet and our society of consumption are not helping the cause much. Far too many of us fall into the trap of purchasing ridiculous fitness products advertised on TV or in the right column of our e-mail browser—you know, like that electrical stimulating belly belt, or ridiculous devices like the Shake Weight or Spin Gym. I'm sorry, but the only calories you'll burn with these rip-offs will happen when you get your credit card statement and your heart rate soars when you realize that you spent actual money on this junk!

The Number on the Scale Doesn't Move Fast Enough

This is a big one, and the hardest for me in particular to acknowledge. I fought the good fight for a long time, saying over and over that it's far better to lose half a pound a week over 20 weeks than to drop 10 pounds in a week. When I first moved to Los Angeles 10 years ago, I started to see just how desperate people were to lose weight *right away*, in the snap of a finger. When my voice of reason and logic failed to penetrate their sense of urgency, I would lose these clients, who would go off to try the latest overnight body-transformation scheme. I saw even more of this desperation when I began to work with women on the talk show *The Revolution*—and, as I've said, I saw the flip side of this desperation as well, which is to say that the ones who lost the most weight right away were the ones most likely to stick with the program, even after the show was over.

I've since accepted the extent to which people get psychologically frustrated when their progress is too slow. You are enduring what feels like Herculean sacrifices to improve your body, but that number on the scale just refuses to budge. So yes, you will inevitably feel discouraged, and you have every right to be frustrated—not only at your body, but at this stupid diet that's making you suffer for no reason. What's the point of depriving yourself of all the foods you love if you have nothing to show for it?

The answer is: THERE IS NO POINT. You *can* get the body you want and deserve without going to hell and back. I'll show you how.

"There are two primary reasons why I failed at other diets: one, they felt like work to me, and two, it always seemed like I was being deprived of the food I really enjoyed. On Harley's program, I always felt satisfied/full. I never felt like I was chained to a diet, but instead, I had simply changed the way I ate. Harley actually taught me how to be much smarter about my food choices, which removed that awful guilt I would feel after every meal. With his simple lifestyle changes, the weight started to drop off pound by pound!"

—Angela Patrick, *lost 8 pounds in 15 days*

CHAPTER

2

Why the Body Reset Will Work

So is there really a diet out there that's actually *good* for our bodies? That works with—instead of against—our bodies' metabolism, that keeps our appetites satiated and our tastebuds entertained, that accommodates our insanely overstuffed schedules while also yielding amazingly fast yet sustainable results? Is there a way to lose weight quickly without risking a trip to the emergency room or guaranteeing that you'll balloon up to an even larger size when it's all over?

Yes, yes, and yes. I've created the Body Reset precisely to help you where all those other diets have let you down. Because trust me, you do NOT have to sacrifice your health or put your life on hold or empty your bank account to finally get the body you've always wanted. You can eat delicious foods, exercise only a few minutes a day, have a huge amount of energy, and feel better than you ever have before, all the while shedding pound after pound after pound.

My plan is completely different from anything you've ever tried before—and *way* more effective. It will help you lose weight right away, and keep that weight off in the years to come. So just stick with me for the next 15 days and I promise that when it's all over your friends won't recognize you. You might not even recognize yourself!

Whatever brought you to pick up this book, *The Body Reset Diet* is going to revolutionize the way you think about dieting—and revolutionize your body in the process. You'll:

- Lose fat quickly and safely
- Experience a big energy boost
- Enjoy improved overall health
- Feel as amazing as you look

Yes, I'll say it again: By the time these 15 days are up, you will look and feel *dramatically* better. And to get there, you won't have to suffer even for a second. You will quickly learn that losing weight is not a form of punishment.

You will also be finding that happy medium on the exercise front—an element of healthy living that most diets either ignore completely or dangerously overemphasize. On *The Body Reset Diet*, you will learn the importance of moving consistently throughout your day for optimum health. It's MUCH more important to move regularly than to throw yourself into some radical exercise regimen that will probably land you in the orthopedist's office before the year's up.

Unlike other diet plans, you will be taking care of your body every step of the way. The secret to *The Body Reset Diet* is that it kick-starts rapid weight loss *without* depleting you of vital nutrients or quality of life. From the very beginning, you'll be getting all the nutrients your body needs to thrive.

There will be no attempts at starving yourself thin here—repeated studies have shown that such efforts inevitably backfire anyway. Five times a day, you'll be filling yourself up with foods that are as satisfying as they are delicious. Even in the first 5 days, you'll never feel hungry because you'll be eating such a high volume of food at regular intervals throughout the day. The food you'll be eating will also be extremely nutrient dense, and your body will be using every calorie you take in.

Grazing versus **Gorging**

Eating just three (or even just two, if you skip breakfast) meals a day isn't good for our blood sugar. Researchers at the University of Toronto found in a study that contrasted the cholesterol and insulin levels of men who ate three large meals a day to those who "nibbled" on 17 meals.[1] Nibbling, or grazing—i.e., eating smaller meals more often—resulted in lower insulin levels, the key to any successful weight-loss plan, and the underlying principle of all my eating protocols. Several other studies support the importance of grazing over gorging to steady our metabolism and increase our body's fat-burning capacities, like one out of Spain that found that teenagers who ate more than four times a day tended to have lower fat levels regardless of exercise habits.[2]

On the Body Reset Diet, you can expect to see rapid weight loss and inches lost within the first 5 days, and this is as much a result of a boosted metabolism as of calorie reduction. Other diets, in contrast, deprive users of various nutrients at the expense of their metabolism. The key to avoiding the seesaw ups and downs of most diets is never to put your body into this self-defeating deprivation mode.

It's critical to understand that we don't lose weight by denying ourselves food, but on the contrary by eating small meals around the clock. Whatever you've been taught, the easiest way to take off the pounds is to eat *more* often, not less. After all, it's when we get really, really hungry that our insulin dips and spikes, which causes our bodies to store food as fat. That's also when we lose sight of our best intentions—and lose control. We end up eating more food than we intended, and certainly more than we needed.

To make your metabolism more efficient than ever, you need to get into the habit of grazing instead of gorging. Eating five times each day on the Body Reset Diet shifts your metabolism into high gear, meaning you'll burn even more calories and shed more fat 24/7—yes, even while you're fast asleep!—without throwing your body into confusion.

The Body Reset Diet will teach you how to maintain consistent blood sugar levels and never experience those dangerous dips in energy that lead to bingeing and general exhaustion and despair. Eating regularly helps tame your appetite, control cravings, and the high amounts of fruits and veggies you'll be consuming will overload you with bioavailable nutrients that unlock your metabolism's true potential.

But perhaps the biggest difference between the Body Reset Diet and the rest of these trendy diets is that my plan is designed for the long haul, to provide guideposts not just for the first 15 days, but for the rest of your life.

Why Diets Fail	Body Reset Solution
The number on the scale doesn't move fast enough.	In the first phase of the Body Reset, you can expect to see rapid weight loss. You'll feel satiated throughout the day and motivated to stick with the plan.
They encourage the false assumption that all calories are created equal.	The Body Reset explains what foods are to be consumed and WHY. By understanding the importance of a high-protein and high-fiber diet, you're empowered to make smarter eating decisions moving forward.
They take up WAY too much time.	It doesn't get easier than throwing raw or frozen ingredients into a blender. It's faster (and much cheaper) than calling for delivery or going out to eat in a restaurant.
The extreme calorie restriction they recommend leads to a state of semi-starvation.	On the Body Reset, you'll consume 3 daily meals and 2 daily snacks made up of protein and fiber that will provide adequate calories and all the nutrients you need to thrive.
They require too many changes at once.	The Body Reset is easy to use and easy to implement, and the changes are incorporated gradually.
They lead to food exhaustion and boredom with a limited range of ingredients, or they require exotic, hard-to-find ingredients.	The Body Reset provides a multitude of delicious, filling recipes that are fun to prepare and consume, and it's built around foods you can buy at any supermarket.
They cost too much.	Once you start blending, you will start saving big money on this diet by using seasonal and/or frozen foods. You'll also save by not eating out in restaurants as much.

Are you ready to get started on the easiest, most rewarding diet you've ever been on?

What You Can Expect to Do on the Body Reset

The Body Reset lasts just 15 days, broken into three distinct 5-day phases. By the end of the 15 days, you may be shocked by how much your body—and your whole perspective on diet and exercise—has changed. You'll:

- Spend less time and money than ever before on food
- Eat more fruits and vegetables than ever before—without even noticing (and trust me, this is coming from someone who *hates* vegetables)
- Prime your metabolism to work with you around the clock
- Give your body access to more fat-burning, usable nutrients than ever before
- Burn fat nonstop all day long (and even while you sleep) without ever setting foot in a gym
- Sculpt your body in just a few minutes a day, with no equipment necessary

What You Can Expect to Learn on the Body Reset

This plan isn't just limited to the next 15 days. A big part of it is about educating you about health and fitness so you'll know why you're eating and moving in this way. The more you understand today, the better you can live tomorrow. I want you to take away more than just a hot body from this book! You'll learn:

How to make the right nutritional decisions. I want you to learn not only *what* is in your meals, but *why* you are eating those particular ingredients in those particular combinations. Why is it so important to eat fiber at every meal? Why is a meal not a meal without a protein and fiber? Why are people who regularly eat fruits and vegetables so much thinner than those who don't? Understanding the difference between good and bad fats, and simple and complex carbohydrates, will empower you to make the right nutritional decisions for the rest of your life.

How to create structure within your day. Instead of eating on the go or grabbing lunch from a vending machine whenever you feel that first stab of hunger (or whenever you feel bored or distracted), you'll learn to schedule the times you eat in advance and to make a ritual out of your meals that allows you to actually enjoy them. And guess what—by planning your meals ahead of time, you'll also save both time and money. You'll be less likely to run out of crucial ingredients, and less likely to order overpriced, greasy takeout at the last minute because you can't think of anything to make that night. Because you'll enter the store armed with a list, you'll be less tempted to fill your cart with unhealthy impulse-item ingredients.

How to become a more efficient eater. Make your calories count. Build your diet around nutrient-dense high volume foods so that your body will adapt to getting more out of less. A blender is one of the best ways to maximize the bioavailability of foods, which is one reason it's the centerpiece of *The Body Reset Diet.* It also happens to be one of the easiest ways to prepare food.

Perhaps most of all, I want you to get it in your head that YOU DO NOT HAVE TO SUFFER TO LOSE WEIGHT!

Like I said: Forget everything you've been told. Weight loss should not be a form of punishment. It is your *reward* for working hard and making the right decisions. It's a real tragedy that, in our all-out apocalyptic struggle to shed the pounds, we've come to regard food as our enemy. Forget that! Food is one of the great pleasures in life, and you *can* eat well and still lose weight; in fact, eating well is the only way *to* lose weight. So let's forget everything we know about nasty "diet food" and bring the joy back into eating again.

Life is difficult enough already. Your diet should be easy—and fun.

CHAPTER

Why Blend?

Before we get into the nitty-gritty details of the three phases, let's talk about the main tool you need to get started: a blender. Most of us have one already, but what do we use it for? Maybe a milkshake every month or so, or perhaps some frozen margaritas when it's hot out.

Well, guess what? This underappreciated kitchen gadget can be an indispensable part of getting you back on the road to wellness (and hotness) again. Learn to love your blender and your body will thank you for it. Blending is one of the quickest, most convenient ways to prepare food. Anyone can do it, on any schedule. You won't have to deal with setting timers or waiting for water to boil; there will be no julienning or defrosting. With a blender, you just throw everything into the jar and press "start," using my guidelines for a complete smoothie. You can create an entire meal in under 90 seconds.

A blender gives you access to a wide range of good-for-you ingredients, putting all sorts of healthy foods at your fingertips. Blending makes the intimidating easy: With the help of a good blender, it's zero effort to get more fruits and vegetables into your diet than you ever thought you could. Blenders are also good tools for disguising what might not be your all-time favorite flavors. For example, you might not like how spinach tastes on its own (I know I'm not the biggest fan), but how about when it's blended with some pears and grapes? You won't even be able to recognize the leafy green superfood; it's the fruit flavors that dominate.

Best of all, your body can actually use these ingredients when they're in blended form, because blenders break down food into molecules that are efficiently metabolized and readily *bioavailable*, i.e., absorbed into

Forever Young:
Fruits and Vegetables

Eating a lot of fruits and vegetables benefits your whole body. Your skin: One recent study suggested that raw veggies might reduce breakouts by as much as 30 percent. Your immune system: Vitamin A, found in carrots, cantaloupe, and lettuce, is known to boost immune system function. And yes, fruits and veggies also promote your eternal youth and beauty: Women who eat a lot of vitamin C–packed foods like oranges and guava have fewer wrinkles than women who don't, according to a recent study that tracked the diets of more than 4,000 American women ages 40 to 74.[1]

your body in a manner that it can use. A 2008 study at the University of Toronto found that certain blenders are capable of disrupting the cell-wall structure of plants and significantly reducing food particle size, which may enhance the bioavailability of essential nutrients in fruits and vegetables. And while this may not be the most appetizing example, a study done with chicken livers measured how blending time impacted the bioavailability of nutrients, in particular iron. The study found that particles processed in a blender for 6 minutes resulted in more than twice the iron of chicken liver blended for just 60 seconds.

Blending versus Juicing

So, you're asking, if blending is so great, isn't juicing better? Juicing takes more time and costs more money, so surely it's healthier—right?

Wrong, wrong, and wrong again. Contrary to conventional wisdom, juicing is *far* inferior to blending, and not just because blenders are infinitely easier to operate and clean than juicers, which also happen to be a headache to assemble and disassemble (and who can possibly keep track of all those parts?).

Juicing also requires a great deal more produce to achieve the same quantity of liquid as an equivalent blended beverage—sometimes three to five times as much. That's because only a small portion of the fruit goes into the finished product of the juice. Have you ever seen how much they throw away at juice bars? They discard all the fibrous parts of the fruit or vegetable that hold all the nutrients.

With blended smoothies, all those nutrients, and the entirety of the fruit or vegetable—including the all-important fiber—are going straight into your body. The waste associated with juicing isn't just a concern from a financial or environmental perspective. It's not doing your body

Choosing the Right **Blender**

Though the first commercial blender wasn't introduced to the market until the 1930s, the concept of a blended beverage is millenia-old—just look at the Indian lassi, a drink of blended fruit and yogurt. These days, blenders are as high-tech as it gets. You can pulverize just about anything in your kitchen, from whole nuts and sesame seeds to full apples and carrots. There are no limits.

When choosing the right blender, here are a few things to consider:

- A minimum of 500 watts, to make sure you have enough power to blend harder produce or nuts. Ideally, you will want even higher than that.
- A large pitcher (that's dishwasher safe), to accommodate smoothies prepared as meal replacements (produce like spinach takes a lot of space)
- A heavy base for stability
- A design that's easy to clean (such as a unit with a flat control panel vs. multiple buttons that's hard to wipe around)
- Capability to grind seeds or cacao beans, etc. (coffee grinders can do this, but you can benefit from it if your blender already can do this)
- On top of these, while not a "must-have," if your blender can also crush ice into a nice "shaved ice" consistency, you can do a lot more with your blender—such as delicious fruit or green cocktails!

Depending on your budget, you can invest in a expensive blender (like Vitamix or Blendtec) or choose from some great budget blenders. My own brand of blender is far more affordable, compares to the higher-end models, and comes with a flat control panel, dishwasher safe parts, and multiple cup sizes to meet your needs. Check it out at bodyresetdiet.com.

My smoothie recipes can be easily modified for all types of blenders. And no matter which you pick, a good blender is a good long-term investment in your health.

any favors, either. Far from being bad for you, the fibrous parts excluded from juices are actually the most nutritious component of the entire plant! As my old professor Dr. Glynn Leyshon at the University of Western Ontario once quipped, "Since most of the nutrients and nearly all of the fiber is in the skin, seeds, and pulp," he said, "you're better off throwing out the juice part and drinking the rest!"

That's right. Once all the fiber has been removed, most juices are left with large and extremely unhealthy quantities of sugar. Some juices have an even higher sugar content—and in many cases more calories—than sugary sodas, and that's saying something. Just think: Making a cup of orange takes the juice of, say, six oranges, and drinking it is much less filling and *way* less nutritious than eating a single orange whole. If you don't believe me, try comparing the nutrient profile of a cup of orange juice (132 calories, 31 grams of carbohydrates, 0.4 gram of fiber, 25 milligrams of calcium, and 64 milligrams of vitamin C) with that of a cup of solid orange segments (82 calories, 19 grams of carbohydrates, 4.5 grams of fiber, 82 milligrams of calcium, and 102 milligrams of vitamin C).

APPLE JUICE VERSUS BLENDED APPLE BEVERAGE

	"Pure" Apple Juice (16 fl oz)	Blended Apple Beverage (16 fl oz)
Calories	240	120
Fat	0 g	0 g
Protein	0 g	0.75 g
Sugar	57 g	19 g
Fiber	0 g	3 g
Cost (approximate)	$2.75	$0.65

Far and away the healthier option of the two—the drink that's lowest in sugar, lowest in calories, highest in protein, and highest in fiber—is the blended apple. All of its nutrients remain intact, and because you're not throwing anything away, the blended apple is also the cheaper option, coming in at only about 32 cents per 8-ounce cup.

The Fiber Factor

Let's look a little more closely at the reasons you should always reach for a blended apple over a juiced one. The most important one bears repeating: because blended drinks, unlike juiced ones, contain both the juice and pulp from your produce, and the pulp contains the number one nutritional benefit of the drink: fiber.

In its natural form, almost every fruit and vegetable has some fiber content, but we don't eat nearly enough produce, and our diets are frighteningly deficient in fiber. The American Dietetic Association recommends women consume a minimum of 25 grams of fiber a day and men consume at least 30 grams, but most Americans get only about 10 grams a day—roughly a third of the recommendations. Ideally, I'd like you to get at least 40 grams of fiber into your daily diet.

More fiber leads to more weight loss; it's just that simple. The vast majority of studies have concluded that more dietary fiber yields greater satiety and lower incidences of hunger: In fact, adding 14 grams of fiber a day has been shown to lead to a 10 percent decrease in caloric intake and an increased weight loss of about 4.2 pounds over a little under 4 months.[2] Another study found that when people increased their intake of soluble fiber by 10 grams a day, their belly fat decreased by 3.7 percent in 5 years, while still another showed that soluble fiber can boost the immune system.[3]

So from now on, you will be eating fiber throughout the day—all five times you eat, in fact. Yes, you might notice that you may need to go to the bathroom more frequently, especially at first, but that's a GOOD thing. The longer food sits in your colon, the more it messes with your blood sugar (and eventually turns to fat). Fiber helps us clear out the intestinal trash that's not doing our bodies any favors.

A Fiber Primer

There are two types of fiber, soluble (meaning it dissolves in water, and is digested by your body) and insoluble (meaning it doesn't dissolve in water, and rather than being digested by your body merely passes through, aiding the digestive process). Both soluble fiber—which is found in seeds, oat bran, lentils, and apples—and insoluble fiber—found in whole grains, vegetables, and beans—passes through our bodies undigested, and both are absolutely essential for maintaining good digestion and fighting a huge range of diseases.

Liquid Energy

Various studies indicate that liquid meals can be more filling than solid meals. *The Body Reset Diet* capitalizes on this science to produce impressive weight-loss results with a combination of smoothies and a high intake of other liquids as well. One study shows that when participants ate a first course of soup before a lunch entrée, they reduced their total calorie intake at lunch (soup + entrée) by an amazing 20 percent, compared to when they did not eat soup. That's one reason you'll be drinking so much water in addition to your smoothies—because a high volume of liquids helps keep your body detoxified and your stomach full.

More **Fiber Facts**

Fiber extends your life span. When the National Cancer Institute and the American Association of Retired Persons (AARP) studied dietary fiber intake in relation to total mortality as well as death from specific causes, they found that both men and women with the highest fiber intake, specifically fiber from whole grains, had a significantly lower risk of death.

Fiber fights disease. A recent study[4] found that diets rich in soluble fiber can help reduce the inflammation that can lead to obesity-related diseases like diabetes and heart disease. The same study found that fiber can help strengthen the immune system.

Fiber keeps your pipes clean. Fiber is perhaps the most important nutrient for maintaining proper bowel health. It bulks up your diet and helps avoid constipation and all the unpleasantness that entails.

Fiber's many health advantages are especially important when it comes to weight loss: first, fiber makes us feel fuller longer, which is a key to curbing cravings. When you drink a cup of juice (which has no fiber), your blood sugar spikes and shortly thereafter dips. The result: Half an hour later, you're already craving yet another cup of juice, an endless supply of still more calories.

This is not the case with fiber-packed blended drinks. Soluble fiber in particular slows the body's absorption of sugar, which steadies the body's insulin levels and prevents those ups and downs that make us so ravenously hungry and lead to such disastrous bingeing. Fiber in beverages, by contrast, can actually make you feel fuller than you would otherwise, a recent study found, as fibrous foods continue to expand in your stomach.[5] The more fiber in the food, the less you will need to feel full: A 2009 study found that people who ate an apple before lunch ate 15 percent fewer calories than those who had applesauce or drank apple juice.[6]

Because fiber keeps us satisfied for so much longer, we tend to eat less and over time, lose more weight. A recent study has shown that fiber consumption can in fact triple weight loss and make us 62 percent less likely to develop diabetes, while a USDA study found that eating 36 grams of fiber a day can prevent your body from absorbing 130 calories a day.[7] Fiber-rich foods are also more calorically dense than low-fiber foods, i.e., high-calorie foods tend to be low in fiber, while low-calorie foods tend to be high in fiber.

Making fiber the centerpiece of your diet is one of the best ways to control your appetite and get more out of every calorie. You'll notice immediately when you start drinking my smoothies that you will NOT feel hungry after you've had one—not 5 minutes later, and not 2 hours later, either. A lot of that is thanks to the high amounts of fiber you'll be eating.

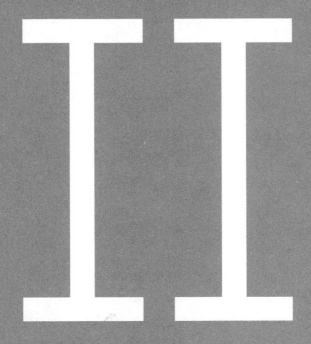

II

The First 15 Days
of the Rest
of Your Life

4

An Overview of the Body Reset

All right, so let's get down to it. First off, as I've already mentioned, throughout these initial 15 days, you'll get into the habit of eating five times daily to maximize the efficiency of your metabolism. Five categories of ingredients, 5 minutes of prep time, five meals daily—that's my highly successful formula.

On the Body Reset, I've even further simplified both the categories of ingredients and the time it takes to make a meal out of them. With the help of a blender, you can make a whole meal in 2 minutes flat, including all prep time. I promise you, there is NO easier way to make amazingly delicious and good-for-you meals, to enjoy either at home or on the go.

Whether you're having a smoothie, a solid meal, or a snack, you will always be eating five times a day, at intervals timed to keep your blood sugar stable and your metabolism at its most efficient.

The Three Phases

The Body Reset Diet is broken up into three distinct 5-day phases lasting a total of 15 days. You'll be alternating nutritious, delicious, and filling smoothies with a number of snacks and meals, all of which you can toss together in 5 minutes max.

Harley's **Reset** Template

You'll:

- Eat five times a day to rev up your metabolism.
- Follow specific nutritional criteria for each meal.
- Build each meal around the same categories of ingredients.
- Prepare each meal in five minutes or less.

After you complete the 15-day kick-start, you will follow a much looser long-term version of this plan. By this point, you'll have learned the benefits of

- Eating five times a day
- Moving consistently from morning till night
- Preparing your own meals

You will also be looking and feeling so good that you'll be motivated to continue this plan on your own. But for the first 15 days, I'm going to hold your hand and tell you exactly what you have to do and why you need to do it.

PHASE I

Diet: In Phase I, between Days 1 and 5, you'll be drinking three smoothies a day and eating two snacks. This period will be the greatest adjustment for your body and brain, but don't worry, this is the reset portion of the Body Reset. The meals are high volume, which means that you'll feel like you are eating a lot of food throughout the entire plan.

Movement: During these first few days, you'll give up your spin class or boot camp and simply walk—a minimum of 10,000 steps a day, a very achievable goal you can track with the help of a pedometer, a tiny device that counts the number of steps you take a day. (Trust me—it will become your favorite new toy! See page 104 for tips on picking out the perfect pedometer.)

PHASE II

Diet: By Phase II, between Days 6 and 10, you'll still be eating five times a day, providing your body with a steady supply of fuel, but now you'll be drinking only two smoothies and having one solid—nonblended, but still healthy, delicious, and extremely easy to prepare—meal a day, plus your usual choice of snacks between the meals.

Movement: In addition to continuing to walk a minimum of 10,000 steps a day, you'll begin a super-simple 5-minute at-home fitness routine 3 days a week to tone your changing body. These exercises will be extremely easy to do and require no equipment, and I'll offer a variety of modifications to suit different fitness levels.

PHASE III

Diet: In Phase III, you'll have just one smoothie a day, plus two meals and two snacks.

Movement: Continue to walk throughout your day until you've logged 10,000 steps. Your strengthening routine will be a slightly extended version of the super-simple resistance exercises I introduced you to in Phase II. In addition to keeping up your regular walking, you'll be alternating between two 5-minute circuits of resistance training 5 days a week. You can do these simple exercises in any room in your house, and with little to no equipment.

	Phase I (5 Days)	Phase II (5 Days)	Phase III (5 Days)
Breakfast	Smoothie	Smoothie	Smoothie
Snack 1	Snack	Snack	Snack
Lunch	Smoothie	Smoothie	Meal
Snack 2	Snack	Snack	Snack
Dinner	Smoothie	Meal	Meal

THE REST OF YOUR LIFE

Diet: You'll still be eating five times a day, but in combinations that you design yourself. You'll have one smoothie a day, two snacks, and two solid meals. And twice a week, you can enjoy "free meals," when you hit the town (or fridge) and eat whatever you want.

Movement: Keep up with the 10,000 steps a day! This I want you to do 7 days a week, 365 days a year, for the rest of your life. This simple modification to your daily habits will transform you from a couch potato to a fit, energetic person—and all you have to do is walk. Five days a week, you'll be doing a slightly increased version of your A and B resistance-training circuits for a total of 10 minutes a day, or less than an hour a week (i.e., less time than you used to spend on a single punitive exercise video).

So there's your cheat sheet—sound pretty simple and straightforward? Trust me, it is.

> "When I was at my heaviest, I thought that I was as comfortable as possible because I gave into every bad craving and let myself rest and relax whenever I wanted to. 'I deserve it,' I told myself. Adjusting to exercise and clean eating was a challenge at first, but as I embraced the uncomfortable and the weight fell off, I felt more alive than I ever have in my whole life. My eyes brightened, my skin got clearer, I slept better, I had enough energy to bounce off the walls, and I had a better sense of structure and discipline to be more productive. I feel healthy now and it's the sexiest, most comfortable feeling ever! And I deserve it!"
>
> —Cherie Nicole, *lost 9 pounds in 15 days*

PHASE

5

Getting Started

Phase I: What You'll Be Doing

You will be eating five times a day: three smoothies and two snacks. You will be walking a minimum of 10,000 steps per day (for easy ways of achieving this goal, see page 105).

What You'll Need
- A blender (see page 26)
- A pedometer (see page 104)
- A shopping list (see page 64)

ASSEMBLING THE SMOOTHIES

The more you know about what's going into your smoothies, the more confident you'll be at substituting similar ingredients from the same categories to add more variety to your drinks later on. First, you need to know that we are NOT talking about those sugar bombs that you get from "healthy" smoothie counters at the food court. Most of those overpriced concoctions are indistinguishable from milk shakes, with a through-the-roof sugar content that will send your appetite spiraling into overdrive and add untold hundreds of calories to your daily intake.

The Body Reset smoothies won't leave you with a massive sugar hangover nor do they taste excessively "healthy." In smoothie making, as in so many other aspects of modern life, the pendulum keeps swinging too far between two extremes: We're either drinking sherbet-stuffed smoothies with 1,800 calories per serving or we're going totally overboard in the opposite direction, blending up jugs of bok choy and red onion for breakfast. I'm sorry, but that's gross. You do NOT have to chug disgusting vegetable-only medleys to lose weight. Food is one of the great pleasures in life, and it should remain so even while you are slimming down.

Forget about both sugary drinks and the kale-stuffed elixirs. This is not a zero-sum game: The Body Reset smoothies are good for your body *and* they taste amazing. They'll steady your blood sugar and curb those all-too-familiar hunger pangs, and they're so satisfying precisely because they all contain the right combination of foods in the right proportions.

And about that: Once you understand the science behind the

ingredients, you'll be able to create an infinite variety of these delicious beverages whenever you want—depending on what's in season or just what mood you're in. Losing weight means combining the right kinds of foods every time you eat. To meet my criteria for a complete meal—one that delivers all the nutrients you need and

Components of the
Perfect Smoothie

- Liquid base (milk, dairy or nondairy; water or flavored water)
- Lean protein (plain nonfat Greek yogurt, protein powder)
- Healthy fat (nuts, seeds, avocado)
- High-fiber carbohydrate (pretty much any fruit or vegetable you can name, though some are better than others; see page 51)

You'll notice that a number of these ingredients overlap—for example, the milk used as the liquid base is also a source of protein, and healthy fats like avocados are also vegetables.

That's why all those stringent (and to my mind ridiculous) food-combining diets—in which you can never eat a carbohydrate at the same meal as a fat, for example—make absolutely no sense to me. Bean-based diets are incredibly healthy, and the nutritional profile of a bean is equal parts carbohydrate, fiber, and fat. And let me tell you, this nation is not getting fat off too many kidney beans!

The key is variety, consuming the widest possible range of foods every time you sit down to eat. My smoothie recipes take all the guesswork out of this balancing act by offering everything you need in one delicious drink.

keeps you craving free until it's time to eat again—each smoothie must contain several predetermined categories of ingredients in addition to the base: a lean protein, a healthy fat, and a high-fiber carbohydrate.

The Case for **Milk**

Dairy products have gotten a bad rap over the past decade, mostly because of their fat content. As with so much of the health "wisdom" we're force-fed, this is nonsense—milk products are among the healthiest foods you can eat!

I'm sure you've heard some well-meaning "expert" argue that humans are the only species who drink milk from another animal—well, so what? We've been doing it for thousands of years. We're also the only species who can fly airplanes and write sonnets and solve physics equations.

Rich in protein, calcium, vitamin D, phosphorus, and other nutrients that have been proven to build your bones and teeth as well as promote the healthy function of your muscles and blood vessels, milk is one of the most perfect foods for the human body. Calcium can help the body switch from fat-storing to fat-burning mode, keeping you slim.

High-calcium foods like milk and yogurt can also directly aid weight-loss efforts. Researchers at the University of Knoxville have found that high-calcium foods, notably dairy sources, have been shown to increase the rate of body fat breakdown and preserve metabolism during dieting.[1] This study also found that eating multiple servings of dairy a day—three or four—can have a much greater effect on weight loss than simply eating calcium supplements or calcium-fortified foods. In another study, participants who consumed the most calcium from dairy products—about 12 ounces of milk a day—consistently lost more weight than those who consumed the least.[2] And there's still more evidence: One recent study found that an ingredient in milk can protect against obesity, while another concluded that dairy-rich products can help people

Ingredient Category #1: Liquid Base

The liquid is the first ingredient you place into the blender when making a smoothie. (A tip for optimal blending is to start with the light ingredients

shed belly fat.[3] Yet another found that women who drank two glasses of milk after weight training were more toned and less fat than women who drank sports drinks.[4]

It's no coincidence that some of the healthiest countries in the world have made dairy products a dietary staple. When I was researching my previous book, *The 5-Factor World Diet*, I was pleased (but not at all surprised) to learn that several of the healthiest countries in the world have dairy-based diets. Svelte Scandinavians often drink a glass of milk with meals, and the French and Greeks both regularly eat yogurt, a fantastic source of the active probiotic cultures we need to keep our immune systems up and running. Many of the smoothies in this book contain Greek yogurt for that very reason—and because it's satisfying and delicious.

As with everything in life, though, not all dairy products have the same nutritional properties. A nonfat plain Greek yogurt will obviously have a different effect on your body than a hunk of Cheddar cheese, precisely because these are extremely different foods that we shouldn't lump together indiscriminately. We'll be sticking with nonfat milk products in our drinks, which give us essential nutrients without weighing us down. And while I don't expect you to replace all of your groceries with organic substitutions, I would recommend buying hormone-free dairy products whenever possible, since the United States is one of the few remaining countries that still permits dairy farmers to use the scary recombinant bovine growth hormone (rBGH) or recombinant bovine somatotropin (rBST) in cows.

and proceed to the heavier ones, though there are no hard-and-fast rules—experiment as you go and figure out what works for you.)

My smoothies generally use either milk or water as a base, though as you get more experienced crafting your own concoctions, you can start to experiment with zero-calorie drinks like naturally sweetened Vitamin Water Zero if you yearn for some extra sweetness. Remember, it's all about making every calorie count, so stick to the simplest liquids to get your smoothie started.

Ingredient Category #2: Lean Protein

Major rule to live by: We need to consume protein *every single time* we eat because it helps us feel full. Forget about a plate of pasta and tomato sauce—that doesn't count as a meal because it doesn't contain protein, one of the three macronutrients used as building blocks of our bodies. High-quality animal sources of protein include chicken, fish, meat, eggs, and dairy; vegetarian sources include whole grains like quinoa and brown rice, legumes like beans and lentils, soy products like tofu, and nuts.

We need protein for numerous reasons: First, unlike carbohydrates or fat, we can't store protein as fat; we must either use it or excrete it, which is why people who eat protein at every meal consistently lose more weight than people who don't. Loading up on protein at breakfast in particular has been shown to be especially effective at reducing food cravings and overeating later in the day.[5]

Protein is also critical for maintaining muscle tissue; a recent study of postmenopausal women on diets found that eating protein throughout the day helped them preserve muscle even as they lost fat—exactly what we're trying to do here![6] Another study confirmed the weight-loss attributes of a high-protein diet, finding that the consumption of protein increases both satiety and the retention of lean muscle mass.[7]

And remember, the more lean muscle tissue you have, the more calories you'll burn throughout the day and night, independent of any physical activity. Just getting enough protein in your diet can help moderate your intake of food and keep obesity at bay.[8] Protein also is important for regulating your resting metabolism (the amount of calories we burn at rest), and it contributes to a feeling of fullness, which is important for curbing hunger between meals.

Ingredient Category #3: Healthy Fat

Some diet books will tell you to shun all fats if you want to lose weight, but in reality, it's not healthy to eliminate fat from our diets altogether.

Fat is, along with protein and carbohydrates, one of the three categories of macronutrients that our bodies need to function. Fat's a major source of energy and a big element in satiety that helps the body absorb vitamins A, D, E, and K. Fat is important for our hormones, nerves, reproductive system, and skin. Our brains need fat, too, especially omega-3 and omega-6 fatty acids, which we can get only through food; the body does not produce these essential nutrients on its own. Most of us get too many omega-6s and not enough omega-3s, so we need to make an effort to reverse that imbalance by favoring omega-3–rich fats in particular.

But though fats are essential, they're not all equally beneficial. There are good fats and bad fats, and we should optimize the levels of "healthy" fats in our diet like those in avocados and almonds while steering clear of the bad fats. If we limit saturated fats (most of which come from animal sources), entirely cut out trans fats (found in processed foods and hydrogenated oils), and up our intake of monounsaturated fats (found in nuts and vegetable oils) and polyunsaturated fatty acids (derived from vegetable sources and fish), we'll be well on our way to getting the body of our dreams.

BAD FATS are broken into two big categories: saturated fats and trans fats. Both saturated fats and trans fats can raise "bad" and lower "good" cholesterol levels and have been linked to heart disease. Saturated fats are mostly found in animal products like red meat, poultry skin, whole milk, butter, and egg yolks, though some vegetable sources such as coconut oil, palm oil, and palm kernel oil also contain high levels. Trans fats, or hydrogenated fats, are for the most part artificial—they're predominantly found in commercially processed food products like doughnuts, cookies, and fried foods—and have zero redeeming qualities. While eating small amounts of saturated fats is unavoidable in most diets, there's absolutely no reason why you should be eating trans fats, period.

GOOD FATS—the fats the Body Reset will focus on—don't raise our total cholesterol. They actually lower our LDL (bad cholesterol) while raising our HDL (good cholesterol). We absolutely must include these good fats as part of a healthy diet. Like the bad fats, the good fats can be grouped into several categories. Monounsaturated fats are found in nuts, avocados, and various vegetable oils, particularly olive oil, which consists of approximately 75 percent monounsaturated fats.

Also critical, especially for brain health, are those polyunsaturated fats found in various fish and vegetable sources, such as flaxseed and chia seeds. Polyunsaturated fats are essential because they provide our bodies with omega-3 fatty acids (or, in the case of the seeds, the omega-3 precursor alpha-linolenic acid, which the body must convert to omega-3). These "good fats" can even help fight Alzheimer's disease and prevent the brain from shrinking.[9] And healthy fats can also improve our skin, hair, nails, and overall appearance. If you eat better, you look better—it's as simple as that.

Ingredient Category #4: High-Fiber Carbohydrates

Though they've gotten a bad rap in recent years, carbohydrates are not at all bad for you. On the contrary, they're one of the most important parts of a healthy diet, and studies show that people who consume at least 50 percent of their calories from carbohydrates are *least* likely to be obese.[10] But as with all foods, there are good carbohydrates and bad carbohydrates, and to lose weight you must understand the difference.

The healthiest carbohydrates—the ones you want to build your diet around—are the ones that rank relatively low on the glycemic index (GI), which is a system that measures the rate at which our blood sugar rises in response to eating certain foods. High-GI foods—like white flour–based breads and pastas or sugary foods (whether those sugars are natural, as in grapes, or less natural, as in licorice)—cause an instant spike in your blood sugar and also in your body's production of insulin. Chronically high levels of insulin are associated with type 2 diabetes, obesity, and even heart disease. Minimizing your sugar intake is absolutely central to losing weight, and not just because of all the calories sugar contains. It's much wiser to choose low-GI carbohydrates that break down slowly, release energy steadily throughout the day, and take much longer to digest.

We also want carbohydrates with a higher fiber content—that crucial ingredient missing not only from juice, but from the white breads and pastas we wolf down with such abandon. Numerous studies have shown that diets high in fiber can achieve weight loss, and the best all-over source of fiber is fruits and vegetables, which not only lower the risk for certain cancers, stroke, heart disease, and high blood pressure but help keep the weight off.[11]

What Else You'll Be Eating

I understand that monotony is the death of many diets—and that texture is an important part of our enjoyment of food—so you'll have two snacks a day even in the first phase of the plan. These snacks are all easily accessible, portable, and require limited preparation. I call these snacks C-snacks for several reasons: because they're for the most part CRUNCHY, which satisfies the very normal desire to chew.

C can also stand for CUT as in cut veggies (everything from celery and carrots to broccoli and zucchini) or fruit. Not all fruit will do, though. Stick to fruit with either edible skin (except grapes) or edible seeds (like berries) or to citrus fruits.

Now, don't get me wrong, I'm not saying that all other fruits are bad for you; not at all. All fruits are good for you, with the nutrients and enzymes our bodies need to flourish—and that's why I include such a wide range of them in the smoothie recipes. However, if you're trying to lose weight fast, stick to the healthier fruits with less sugar and more fiber that will promote faster weight loss in the first 15 days.

SNACK FRUITS

Eat More...		Than...	
Apples	Berries	Mangoes	Cantaloupes
Pears	Cherries	Papayas	Honeydew melons
Peaches	Kiwifruit	Bananas	Watermelons
Nectarines	Oranges	Grapes	
Plums		Pineapples	

You can also eat CRACKERS with a high fiber content; check the label and make sure there are more than 5 grams of fiber per 100 calories. Some of my favorite brands are Finn Crisp, Ryvita, Wasa, and Kavli.

Another major detail about these snacks: As with any meal, they MUST be eaten with a protein! Fruit alone is not enough. Carrots on their own might be "healthy," but they are not a complete snack. Quite often, eating these alone can make you even hungrier.

This is nonnegotiable, because a meal is not a meal and a snack is not a snack unless there's protein and fiber involved, so *every* time you sit down to eat make sure you include both. That means crackers on their own aren't enough; you must combine them with a dip (made from nonfat Greek yogurt seasoned with onion soup or ranch mix) or maybe some hummus or a low-fat bean dip.

All of the snacks should be about 150 calories and contain at least 5 grams of fiber, 5 grams of protein, and *less* than 10 grams of sugar.

A few examples of some easy combinations you can try:

• Celery with almond butter

• Whole grain crackers with hummus

• Carrots with onion dip (made from nonfat Greek yogurt and onion soup mix)

Popcorn

It's a great idea to keep some low-fat popcorn around the house for a delicious snack in a hurry. My favorite brand is Naked: A 150-calorie serving contains approximately 6 grams of fiber, 5 grams of protein, and 4 grams of fat. The Whole Foods 365 brand is also a great low-fat popcorn, and there are several other good microwaveable varieties as well. Of course, if you really want to make a habit of eating this healthy snack, I suggest you buy an air popper for about $15 and just pop whole kernels. The popcorn tastes fresher, and your machine will pay for itself in just a few months.

- Lowfat popcorn^{**+}

- Roasted soy nuts^{**}

- Snack bars^{**+} (try Shaklee or Vega)

- Freeze-dried green peas (try the ones sold under Target's Archer Farms label)

- Chickpea snacks^{**+} (I like the ones made by Good Bean)

- Apple with fat free cheese

- Pear and sliced lean turkey

- Cucumber and smoked salmon

- Crackers and almond butter

- High-protein, high-fiber cereal (e.g., Kashi Go Lean, Optimum Blueberry Cinnamon)^{**+}

- Boiled edamame^{**}

** *These foods already contain both fiber and protein so can be eaten as stand-alone snacks.*

+ *Snack bars, cereals, and other prepackaged snacks must meet the basic nutritional requirements of the rest of your C-snacks: They must have no more than 150 calories and contain at least 5 grams of fiber, 5 grams of protein, and less than 10 grams of sugar.*

For serving sizes, nutrition information, recommended brands and products, and a more comprehensive list of snacks, see page 179.

What Else You'll Be Drinking

In addition to the smoothies, you need to drink a steady supply of other liquids throughout the day. Water in particular helps you flush out toxins from your body that might be dragging you down and keeping your weight higher than it needs to be.

Drinking helps fill you up and increases satiety, and keeping enough

liquid in your body is essential for staying in good shape. Dehydration brings bad side effects, including fatigue, headaches, and muscle cramping—all symptoms that might very easily be mistaken for hunger. So the next time you think you're hungry, have a tall glass of water first, and your growling stomach just might quiet down.

For the duration of the Body Reset (and, come to think of it, for the duration of your time on earth), I want you to be drinking *3 to 4 liters of fluids a day*, which might sound like a lot, but trust me, your body will soon grow to love it. Drinking lots of liquids keeps your body clean and detoxed, and it tricks your stomach into feeling fuller than it actually is.

ACCEPTABLE BEVERAGES

Water

The mother of all drinks is water, and I want you to be getting a lot of it every day—around 3 liters if you're a woman and 4 liters if you're a man. And yes, that's a suggested *minimum*. There are lots of different ways you can get your fill of water:

Flat water: My favorite brand of bottled water is Smartwater, but regular tap water always does the trick. You can also invest in a water filter like those made by Brita or PUR for your home.

Sparkling water: You can buy sparkling water like San Pellegrino or Perrier, or you can make your own at home with Sodastream soda makers (www.sodastreamusa.com), which cost as little as $80 and can save you big bucks long term.

Flavored ice cubes or flavored water: If you want to add some subtle flavor to either still or sparkling water, I'm a big fan of making flavored ice cubes. To do this, just take the grated peel of an orange or lemon, put it in ice cube tray, and add water. A few hours later, add a few ice cubes to your water for a delicious twist.

You can also add a wedge of fruit or a cucumber slice directly to your water.

Sugar-Free Drinks

If you occasionally feel the need for something a little more flavorful than water, there are quite a few delicious drinks out there you can try. (But let me emphasize that these should be in *addition* to water, not instead of it.) Some of my favorites include Fuze Slenderize, Vitaminwater Zero, and when I exercise in the heat, Powerade Zero. You can also use these, as I've mentioned, to spice up your smoothie bases without adding any extra calories.

Coffee/Coffee Drinks

I am a huge fan of caffeine and in fact spent 3 years as a caffeine scientist for the Canadian Department of National Defense, so I know what I'm talking about when I say caffeine can be a great addition to your diet. As long as you aren't adding any caloric sweeteners or full-fat dairy to your coffee, which is naturally calorie free, I encourage you to keep drinking and enjoying your favorite caffeinated beverages. In fact, I don't understand why any diet books ever advise otherwise. So many cleanses have you remove all caffeinated beverages from your diet, but why? Caffeine is a proven appetite suppressant and it provides much-needed energy, so why would you ever eliminate your morning coffee when it's both good for you and completely delicious?

Coffee in particular contains powerful antioxidants that might prevent the development of type 2 diabetes and reduce risk factors associated with heart disease and strokes.[12] Coffee drinking could reduce our risk of developing both endometrial and skin cancers, and frequent coffee consumption has also been linked to lower rates of Parkinson's disease and Alzheimer's disease.[13] Even decaf can sharpen our memories and lower our chance of developing diabetes.[14] And a recent study

even found that coffee drinkers live longer than everyone else, so drink up—provided you skip all the nasty additives we've become so fond of dumping in our coffees.[15] Stick with black coffee or espresso; you do not want to be getting any of your calories in liquid form.

Coffee is also a great source of energy. To keep the weight off, we need to get moving (which is much easier said than done when we're laid low by another caffeine-withdrawal migraine—thanks, but no thanks). Of course, as in all things, moderation is key. Too much caffeine can keep you awake, and multiple studies have shown that chronic sleep deprivation makes you fatter. So drink enough caffeine to keep you going—but not too late so that it keeps you awake all night.

Tea

Tea is another deliciously versatile beverage that can also be an indispensable diet aid. It's the second most popular drink in the world, outpaced only by water. And though many Americans drink tea regularly, they all too often dump large quantities of sweeteners in it. The same old story . . .

But in its purest form, tea is naturally calorie free. Though all teas come from the same source, different processing methods have produced a range of different varieties, all of which contain different quantities of caffeine and have slightly different health properties. One thing they all have in common: They might help us lose weight. A recent study[16] out of Kobe University in Japan found that regular consumption of tea can counteract the fattening effect of junk food, so drink up.

Experiment with the whole range of teas and find the one you like:

Black tea, which has the most caffeine (though still less than coffee), contains antioxidants known as polyphenols and has weight-loss properties. A 2001 Boston University study found that drinking black tea can help reduce a symptom of coronary artery disease.[17]

Green tea and **white tea**, both of which have less caffeine than black and oolong teas, have extremely powerful antioxidant properties that can protect against cancer and heart disease, and both teas can also lower bad cholesterol levels. Green tea in particular might also be a useful weight-loss aid. It's been shown to stabilize blood sugar and reduce people's risk of developing type 2 diabetes. In one study, diabetic rats given green tea lost significantly more weight and had much lower cholesterol levels than those not treated with the tea.[18] Another recent study, on mice, found that even in conjunction with a high-fat diet green tea can help keep off the pounds.[19]

Oolong tea, a type of green tea, slightly lower on the caffeine scale, is chock-full of polyphenols and catechins, antioxidants renowned for their anti-inflammatory qualities. Oolong tea might also help regulate blood sugar and increase metabolism by 10 percent for 2 hours after drinking. Several recent studies found that oolong tea might be an effective obesity treatment, and that regular consumption of oolong tea can lead to weight loss and an improved metabolism.[20]

Herbal teas are generally caffeine free and are made from a great variety of ingredients, everything from fruits to seeds (and sometimes not any tea leaves), though I wouldn't place any big bets on all those "slimming teas" that have cropped up in health food stores in recent years (and I certainly wouldn't recommend that you embark on one of those tea-only cleanses that has users chug gallons of milk thistle every day).

Other Drinks

I'd like you to eliminate all other beverages from your diet, at least for the first 15 days. As we move into the "rest of your life" phase, you'll be allowed some latitude in the occasional glass of red wine (or more at one of your biweekly free meals), but for now, let's just stick with the basics of water and calorie-free drinks like coffee and tea. I'm not saying you can't ever have alcohol again—by no means—but its sky-high sugar content disqualifies it from the reset portion of our plan. So for the next 15 days, just say no—then we'll talk about alcohol.

What Results Can You Expect to See?

According to the USDA's Economic Research Service (ERS), the average American consumed between 2,600 and 2,800 calories per day between 2003 and 2009, but because it's difficult to estimate calorie consumption accurately, the USDA predicts that daily calorie consumption is actually higher than this already-staggering figure.[21] Even more depressing: A report published in the *Journal of Food Composition and Analysis* revealed that Americans get one-third of their calories from junk foods like soft drinks, sweets, desserts, alcoholic beverages, and salty snacks.[22] No wonder we're so fat!

The good news is that if you press the reset button and change the way you eat for just these first 5 days, you will see immediate, and dramatic results. Just look at the following chart if you don't believe me!

Based on the chart on the next page, if your eating habits even vaguely resemble those of the "average American," you can expect to start dropping the pounds *immediately* on the Body Reset. Instead of empty calories that stimulate your appetite without

	Average American Diet (calories)	Phase I Body Reset Diet (calories)
Breakfast	Bowl of cereal with 2% milk (400) Grande 2% latte (190) 590	– White smoothie (302)
Snack 1	Bottle of "pure" orange juice (240)	Veggies with almond butter (150)
Lunch	Bottle of soda (150) Foot-long BLT sub with mayo and cheese (720) 870	– Red smoothie (317)
Snack 2	Candy bar (320)	Low-fat popcorn (110)
Dinner	Chicken wings (400) Mashed potatoes (250) Green beans (100) 750	– Green smoothie (292)
Total Calories Consumed	**2,770**	**1,211**

benefiting your body in any way, you'll be filling up with large amounts of protein and fiber designed to keep you feeling energetic and craving free all day and night. Even if you don't eat like the average American in the chart above, you may be consuming extra calories without realizing it. All you have to do is make the decision to lose the weight, and the pounds will come flying off.

What If You **Don't** Have a **Blender?**

We don't always have fresh produce and blenders available to us. But we can't use this as an excuse to fall off the wagon. When I'm in a jam, I like to use meal replacements (MRPs). These have all the essential components of the smoothie meals, including high-quality protein, fiber, healthy fat, and micronutrients. They come in two forms: powdered and liquid. The liquid form is conveniently available at most grocery stores and usually comes in a few flavors. Meal replacements also come in the powdered form and can be made simply by adding water. I prefer powder most of the time because it's easier to keep on hand when I'm traveling. It fits in your desk, your purse, even your pocket. It's slightly more cost effective, and you can customize it by adding additional ingredients if you want to add extra nutrients or flavors in the form of fruits, vegetables, or or healthy fats. Shaklee 180 makes a great meal replacement. It has everything you need, tastes great, and is super convenient.

CHAPTER 6

Making the Smoothies

All right, now let's get down to the serious business of actually making the meals that you'll enjoy over the next 15 days. You'll enjoy a white smoothie for breakfast, a red one for lunch, and a green one for dinner, but you can interchange them as you please—as long as you're getting all three of them in the first 5 days.

The first rule I followed in coming up with these recipes is to be adaptable above all else. I know everyone's tastes differ, so for all of my smoothies, I offer slight and not-so-slight variations to suit a wide range of tastes, and to keep your palate entertained—after all, boredom has

Watch Your **Portions**

One more important note: If you're a man or a woman who weighs more than 175 pounds, you need to increase the serving sizes by one-third to get all the nutrition and energy you need. In the three main smoothie recipes, I'll offer modifications in portion size to get you started. If you drop below 175 pounds over the course of this plan, then adjust your portion sizes accordingly.

been the death of many diets. It's important that you love what you're eating, so if apples aren't for you, toss in a pear instead.

If you don't like the apples in the white smoothie, then swap in peaches, and swap in cinnamon for the vanilla. Following each of the basic three smoothie recipes is a chart with suggestions for substitutions. Mix and match and see what pleases your tastebuds. The important thing is that you find recipes that keep you coming back for more. By the time you're finished with this plan, you'll be an expert at building your own smoothies with whatever you've got in the house.

STEP 1: MAKE YOUR SHOPPING LIST

Please, don't go to the grocery store on an empty stomach! And if you do, at least try to avoid the aisles with the most tempting foods if you don't think you'll be able to resist them.

The evening before you begin Phase I, buy all the ingredients you need to get through your first 5 days with ease. Remember, to avoid the pitfalls of yo-yo dieters, advance preparation is critical. I promise you, if you stick to this plan, you will NOT be hungry. But still, don't put yourself in a situation w   u don't have the right ingredients for your lunch smoothie and so decide, just this once, to grab a quick cheeseburger instead. That's not going to fly, especially not during Phase I! Stock your pantry with the following foods so that you'll have everything you need in advance to stay on track.

Produce

5 red apples

5 small bananas

3 oranges

1 bag red or green grapes

5 pears

2 avocados

10 cups spinach

3 limes

Frozen Items

4 bags frozen raspberries

2 bags frozen blueberries

Other

Ground cinnamon

Almonds or almond meal, depending on the strength of your blender

Plain or vanilla protein powder (see page 176 for a complete guide to buying protein powder)

Ground or whole flaxseeds or chia seeds, depending on the strength of your blender (Some, like the Vitamix or Blendtec, will be able to grind the seeds themselves. Less powerful machines might require preground seeds.)

Dairy

½ gallon fat-free organic milk (or nondairy milk of your
    preference)

1 quart fat-free plain Greek yogurt (Chobani, Oikos, Fage,
    Trader Joe's)

Drinks

Coffee, tea

Water

Vitaminwater Zero (or whatever you'd like, as long as it's calorie free)

Don't Wait: Start **Today!**

Clients and readers often ask me what's the best day to start a diet, and I always have the same answer: today. The best time to start a diet is right now! But since you probably don't have some of the ingredients necessary to get going, you might need to do some advance planning.

What's the beginning of your weekly cycle? For people who work Monday through Friday, I often recommend starting on a Saturday. You hit the grocery store Friday after work with your shopping list, then you wake up on Saturday and start blending. Over the weekend, you'll have more time to focus on perfecting your smoothies and adjusting to your new diet. By the time Monday rolls around, you'll already be on Day 3, or almost halfway through Phase 1. Because you'll have momentum, and the confidence that comes with 2 days of smoothie making under demands of your workweek catch up with you. But like I said—any day is a good day, as long as it's soon. The important thing is getting started!

A **Rainbow** of Good Health

As with any food, there's a strong aesthetic component to the perfect smoothie, with those little stripes of orange and green and white all blended into a beautiful spiral. This pleasing appearance might stimulate your enjoyment of your drink, or so believe the Japanese, who think that a good meal should stimulate all five senses, including sight. The Japanese concept of *goshiki* states that every meal should have at least five colors: white (rice, tofu, or fish); yellow (scrambled eggs or squash); red or orange (carrots or sweet potatoes); green (any green vegetable you want!); and black, dark purple, or brown (eggplant or seaweed). *Goshiki* ensures that a meal will please both the eyes *and* the palate— and in the process hit the main categories of ingredients that make up a well-balanced meal. We've pretty much lost this concept in North America, but I still believe that the aesthetics of a meal influence our enjoyment of it.

These colors have an important nutritional purpose, too. To bypass the boredom induced by most diets, which have you eat the same foods over and over, we've placed an emphasis not only on the macronutrients—the fiber, the healthy fats, and so on—but also on the micronutrients, and that's where the colors come in. Red foods are high in nutrients like cancer-fighting lycopene, while orange and yellow foods contain carotenoids, which boost the immune system and reduce heart disease risk. Blue foods are antioxidant powerhouses, and white foods, in addition to being a great source of potassium, might also reduce cancer risk. Green foods, of course, have endless benefits, as they contain everything from folates to lutein. So remember: Colorful food doesn't just look good; it also has a direct impact on your health. To get the full range of nutrients you need, you should be consuming a whole rainbow of foods each and every day.

Snacks

When it comes to snacks, you're free to choose any protein and fiber
nutrient-rich snack that doesn't exceed 150 calories (for women) or
200 calories (for men). Make sure there's at least 5 grams protein,
5 grams fiber, and has no more than 5 grams fat or 10 grams of
sugar. Refer to page 179 for a list of suggested snacks and choose
several that you'll want to enjoy in the first 5 days. I'd pick up a
pound of turkey, a package of edamame, some Ryvita crackers, a
bag of baby carrots, and some hummus. Also get some extra fruits
and finger-food veggies just in case. Whatever you do, just make
sure you have enough snacks for 5 whole days so that you don't go
running to the vending machine.

STEP 2: SET A SCHEDULE

Starting today, you will be eating five times a day, every day, so to avoid
getting too hungry, I want you to sit down and figure out in advance when
exactly you'll be having your three smoothies and two snacks. I want your
first day on the plan to be a total success, so I really recommend you do
this either the night before you begin, or early in the morning of Day 1.

Figure out times that work with your schedule, when you can realis-
tically sit down and take 15 minutes for yourself. I like to eat at 7 a.m.,
10 a.m., 1 p.m., 4:15 p.m., and 7:30 p.m. If it's easier to start on the weekend, when you have more control over your schedule, then by all means
do that. Allow yourself the focus you need. The important thing is that
you space these meals and snacks consistently so that you don't get too
hungry and lose your resolve. Plan meal and snack times ahead so that
your body will adapt to these intervals and know what to expect. It's all
about conditioning from the inside on out.

For an example of a Phase I schedule, please see page 106.

STEP 3: MAKE THE SMOOTHIES

Now that you have everything you need on hand, it's time for your first meal!

Build Your Own Smoothie

And now for the ultimate mix and match of smoothie making!

You can exercise a lot of creativity when it comes to making smoothies—any and all fruits and vegetables are acceptable as long as the overall profile of the meal fits our fiber and protein goals. So pick an ingredient from each of the following categories and blend away!

Ingredient Category

- Liquid base
- Protein
- Healthy fat
- High–fiber carbohydrate

INGREDIENT CATEGORY #1: LIQUID BASE
Choose One:

Water (add as much as you prefer in your smoothies)

Water, Flavored

Fuze Slenderize

Powerade Zero

Vitaminwater Zero

Milk, Dairy
Fat-free or 1% milk (¾ cup maximum)

Milk, Nondairy (¾ cup maximum)
Almond milk
Hemp milk
Oat milk
Rice milk
Soy milk

INGREDIENT CATEGORY #2: PROTEIN
Choose One

Protein Powder
Brown rice
Dairy (whey or casein)
Egg white
Pea
Soy

Tofu (I like soft regular or silken tofu)

Yogurt
Fat-free Greek yogurt
Fat-free regular yogurt

INGREDIENT CATEGORY #3: HEALTHY FAT
Choose One

Avocado

Nuts
Almonds

Cashews

Macadamia nuts

Walnuts

Peanuts (officially a legume, but we'll group it in nuts)

Seeds

Chia seeds (always add right before consuming)

Flaxseeds

Pumpkin seeds, raw, unsalted

Sunflower seeds, raw, unsalted

INGREDIENT CATEGORY #4: HIGH-FIBER CARBOHYDRATE
Choose One

Fruits

While pretty much anything goes when it comes to fruits and vegetables, you should know that certain fruits have more fiber than others. Blackberries and raspberries, for example, are incredibly high in fiber, while bananas and melons are not. I'm by no means saying that you can't put bananas in your smoothies, but if you do, you also need an additional fiber source like chia seeds (which is also a healthy fat) or psyllium to meet the required nutritional profile. So if you're making a piña colada smoothie, you need to make adjustments to compensate for the low fiber profile of both pineapples and bananas.

HIGHEST-FIBER FRUITS

Blackberries	1 cup	8 g
Raspberries	1 cup	8 g
Pear	1 medium, with skin	6 g
Orange	1 medium	4 g
Apple	1 medium, with skin	4 g
Blueberries	1 cup	4 g

Speaking of piña colada smoothies: Certain fruits are also more calorically dense than others. You are absolutely permitted to eat them, but again, you'll have to make certain adjustments, principally when it comes to yield. Your piña colada smoothie will be somewhat smaller than your apple pie smoothie, since gram for gram, a banana is twice as calorically dense as an apple with only half the fiber. A smoothie built around raspberries or blackberries, on the other hand, is both high in fiber and low in sugar, so your serving size can be a bit larger.

HIGHEST-SUGAR FRUITS

Mango	1 cup	30 g
Red seedless grapes	1 cup	25 g
Papaya	1 cup	20 g
Banana	1 medium	20 g

LOWEST-SUGAR FRUITS

Cranberries	1 cup, raw	4 g
Raspberries	1 cup	5 g
Blueberries	1 cup	14 g
Grapefruit	1 cup	16 g

Vegetables

The sky's the limit when it comes to veggies, except when it comes to fat-based veggies like avocados and olives. I'm not saying they're bad—by no means—but for our purposes they belong with the healthy fats, not the high-fiber carbohydrates, and should be used sparingly.

The vegetables that blend best in smoothies are leafy greens. In our green smoothie, we got you started with our champion of champions, spinach, which has a mild taste but still delivers all the amazing health benefits of these vegetables. As always, though, I recommend you walk before you run—i.e., go for gentler spinach and lettuces before trying Swiss chard and kale.

Leafy Greens

Spinach

Kale

Lettuce and salad greens (romaine, arugula, rocket, etc.)

Swiss chard

Watercress

Other leafy greens (collards, mustard greens, bok choy, beet greens)

Other Good Vegetables

Broccoli

Cucumber

Radicchio

Other Flavor Accents

Cinnamon

Ginger

Herbs (basil, mint)

Lemon

Lime

Vanilla

Smoothie Recipes

BREAKFAST

White Smoothie

Serves 1

TIPS:
- Be sure to leave the skin on the apple for the fiber boost.
- It's also a good idea to buy a couple of extra bananas, peel them, and throw them in the freezer for future smoothies.
- Smoothies blend faster if you add liquid first. If you like your drinks thinner, feel free to add ice cubes or cold water. This is a great way to increase the volume without adding to your caloric load.

Ingredients

5	raw almonds, whole or chopped
1	red apple, unpeeled, cored and chopped
1	small banana, frozen and cut into chunks
¾	cup fat-free plain Greek yogurt
½	cup fat-free milk
½	teaspoon ground cinnamon, or to taste

In a blender or food processer, blend the almonds until finely ground. (If your blender isn't powerful enough to grind almonds, you can buy chopped almonds or even almond meal instead.) Add the apple, banana, yogurt, milk, and cinnamon. Blend until of desired consistency.

Nutrition Info
Calories: 325
Total Fat: 4 grams
Carbs: 56 grams
Protein: 19 grams
Fiber: 8 grams

Modified Version (if you weigh more than 175 pounds)

7   raw almonds

1⅓   red apple, unpeeled, cored and chopped

1⅓   small banana, frozen and cut into chunks

1   cup fat-free plain Greek yogurt

¾   cup fat-free milk

¾   teaspoon ground cinnamon, or to taste

Nutrition Info
Calories: 415
Total Fat: 5 grams
Carbs: 70 grams
Protein: 25 grams
Fiber: 11 grams

SUBSTITUTIONS

Base Fruit	Accent Flavor
Apple	Cinnamon, to taste
Pear	Ginger, to taste
Peach	Vanilla, to taste

Why These Ingredients?

I devised these recipes with the goal of helping you not only lose weight but improve your overall health. Every main ingredient has some important health qualities. See Appendix A, page 171, for a breakdown of the main ingredients in all three colors of smoothies, and an explanation of why they will work wonders on your body.

LUNCH

Red Smoothie

Serves 1

Although nothing beats fresh berries for a snack, frozen fruit is an essential standby for making frosty smoothies year-round. Flash-frozen fruit has the same nutrients as fresh fruit, as long as you choose brands that have no added sugar. (Most don't.) Feel free to mix up your berry choices—strawberries and blackberries work just as well. Make sure to use ground flaxseeds rather than whole flaxseeds unless you have a strong enough blender, which will grind up the seeds for you.

TIP: You can make this smoothie ahead of time if you prefer: Blend it in the morning, pour the smoothie into a shaker bottle, and take it along with you to work. Store in the refrigerator until ready to serve. Add ice as desired and shake well before serving.

Ingredients

1   cup frozen raspberries

¼   cup frozen blueberries

½   orange, peeled

1   scoop vanilla protein powder

1   tablespoon ground flaxseeds (or whole flaxseeds, depending on your blender)

In a blender or food processor, combine the raspberries, blueberries, orange, protein powder, and flaxseeds. Blend until of desired consistency.

Nutrition Info
Calories: 271
Total Fat: 5 grams
Carbs: 43 grams
Protein: 27 grams
Fiber: 11 grams

Modified Version (if you weigh more than 175 pounds)

1⅓ cups frozen raspberries

½ cup frozen blueberries

½ orange, peeled

1⅓ scoops vanilla protein powder

1½ tablespoons ground flaxseeds

¾ cup cold water

Nutrition Info
Calories: 325
Total Fat: 7 grams
Carbs: 55 grams
Protein: 36 grams
Fiber: 14 grams

SUBSTITUTIONS

BASE FRUIT	FIBER/HEALTHY FAT	PROTEIN
Blueberries/Raspberries	Flaxseeds	Vanilla protein powder
Strawberries	Chia seeds	Other flavor protein powder
Blackberries	Ground walnuts	Fat-free Greek yogurt

DINNER

Green Smoothie

Serves 1

*This is a great way to add leafy greens to your diet.
Here, spinach is paired with sweet grapes and pears,
creamy yogurt and avocado, and a splash of lime juice.
For best flavor, select a ripe pear for this recipe.*

TIP: Since you are using only part of the avocado, store
the remainder for your next two rounds of green smoothies.
Carve out a slice, then tightly cover the leftover avocado
in plastic wrap and refrigerate until you need it again. It will
keep for several days in the fridge.

Ingredients

- 2   cups spinach leaves, packed
- 1   ripe pear, unpeeled, cored and chopped
- 15   green or red grapes
- ³⁄₄ cup fat-free plain Greek yogurt
- 2   tablespoons chopped avocado
- 1–2 tablespoons fresh lime juice

In a blender or food processor, combine the spinach, pear, grapes, yogurt,
avocado, and lime juice. Blend until of desired consistency.

Nutrition Info
Calories: 275
Total Fat: 6 grams
Carbs: 48 grams
Protein: 20 grams
Fiber: 9 grams

Modified Version (if you weigh more than 175 pounds)

2½ cups spinach leaves, packed

1½ ripe pears, unpeeled, cored and chopped

20 green or red grapes

1 cup fat-free plain Greek yogurt

2½ tablespoons chopped avocado

2 tablespoons fresh lime juice, or to taste

Nutrition Info

Calories: 315

Total Fat: 8 grams

Carbs: 65 grams

Protein: 27 grams

Fiber: 12 grams

SUBSTITUTIONS

Vegetable	Fruit	Healthy Fat	Protein	Sweetener
Spinach	Pear	Avocado	Greek yogurt	Grapes
Kale	Apple	Almonds	Silken tofu	Frozen pineapple
Baby arugula	Banana	Walnuts	Fat-free milk	
Romaine lettuce		Chia seeds		

Congratulations! You've just completed your first day of Phase I—and you've learned how to make simple, nutritious meals for the rest of your life. You'll find all the smoothie recipes you need starting on page 76.

> "As a working mom of four kids (two of them with special needs), I would LOVE to tell other busy women that weight loss and health are just around the corner for them if they want them badly enough. They just need to take it one day at a time and realize that taking care of themselves is NOT selfish. On the contrary, it's the most loving gift they can give to their loved ones. If I can do it with all my time constraints (and my own physical limitations), then anyone can!"
>
> —Mercedes Johnson, *lost 13 pounds in 15 days*

MORE SMOOTHIE RECIPES

WHITE SMOOTHIES

Apple Pie Smoothie   Serves 1

Be sure to leave the skin on the apple for the added fiber. It's a good idea to buy a couple of extra bananas and throw them in the freezer for future smoothies.

TECHNIQUE TIP: Smoothies blend faster if you add both the fruit and the liquid or yogurt at the same time. If you like your drinks thinner, feel free to add ice cubes or cold water.

- 5   raw almonds
- 1   red apple, unpeeled, cored and chopped
- 1   small frozen banana, chopped
- 6   ounces fat-free plain Greek yogurt
- ½   cup fat-free milk
- ½   teaspoon ground cinnamon, or to taste

In a blender or food processor, blend the almonds until finely ground. Add the apple, banana, yogurt, milk, and cinnamon. Blend until of desired consistency.

Nutrition Info
Calories: 325
Total Fat: 4 grams
Carbs: 56 grams
Protein: 19 grams
Fiber: 8 grams

White Peach Ginger Smoothie

Serves 1

Remember, the riper the fruit, the sweeter the smoothie. If peaches are in season, select the ripest you can find at the market. If not, use frozen peaches.

SERVING TIP: Just for fun, the raspberries aren't blended in this drink. Instead, they are dropped into the glass; serve this drink with a spoon for scooping up the berries.

2	peaches, pits removed and chopped
6	ounces fat-free plain Greek yogurt
2	tablespoons fresh lime juice
½	teaspoon finely chopped peeled fresh ginger or pinch of ground ginger
½	cup fresh raspberries
10	deshelled pistachios, crushed or coarsely chopped (unsalted)

In a blender or food processor, combine the peaches, yogurt, lime juice, and ginger. Blend until of desired consistency. Pour into a tall serving glass. Gently stir in the raspberries and garnish with the pistachios.

Nutrition Info
Calories: 300
Total Fat: 2 grams
Carbs: 41 grams
Protein: 27 grams
Fiber: 9 grams

Tropical Morning Smoothie

Serves 1

Greek yogurt provides almost double the protein of regular yogurt. That and its super-creamy texture make it an ideal addition to a healthy smoothie. However, if you can't find it, feel free to substitute fat-free milk, almond milk, or soy milk.

SHOPPING TIP: Opt for fresh pineapple over canned pineapple for this recipe.

- 1/2 cup fresh or frozen mango chunks
- 1/2 cup fresh pineapple chunks
- 1 frozen banana, chopped
- 6 ounces fat-free plain Greek yogurt
- 2 tablespoons ground flaxseeds

In a blender or food processor, combine the mango, pineapple, banana, yogurt, and flaxseeds. Blend until of desired consistency

Nutrition Info
Calories: 300
Total Fat: 6 grams
Carbs: 38 grams
Protein: 22 grams
Fiber: 8 grams

Pear Spice Smoothie Serves 1

This drink is especially good in the fall, when pears are ripe.

SHOPPING TIP: Experiment with the different types of protein powders now available at the market. Once you've found one you like, you can save money by purchasing a big container.

- 1 pear, unpeeled, cored and chopped
- 1 frozen banana, chopped
- 1 teaspoon finely chopped peeled fresh ginger or pinch of ground ginger

  Pinch of ground cinnamon

  Pinch of ground nutmeg
- 2 tablespoons vanilla or unflavored protein powder
- ½ cup ice cubes or chips

In a blender or food processor, combine the pear, banana, ginger, cinnamon, nutmeg, protein powder, and ice. Blend until of desired consistency.

Nutrition Info
Calories: 300
Total Fat: 2 grams
Carbs: 55 grams
Protein: 25 grams
Fiber: 10 grams

Fall Fruit Frosty

Serves 1

The familiar flavors of this mild smoothie will please the whole family.

SHOPPING TIP: Greek yogurt is often sold in 6-ounce containers. If you make a lot of smoothies, you can certainly buy a bigger container and use ¾ cup (equal to 6 ounces) for this recipe.

1	green apple, unpeeled, cored and chopped
1	ripe green pear, unpeeled, cored and chopped
6	ounces fat-free plain Greek yogurt
2	teaspoons peanut butter
1	cup small ice cubes or chips

In a blender or food processor, combine the apple, pear, yogurt, peanut butter, and ice. Blend until of desired consistency.

Nutrition Info
Calories: 300
Total Fat: 4 grams
Carbs: 52 grams
Protein: 18 grams
Fiber: 10 grams

RED SMOOTHIES

Ruby Red Frostie

Serves 1

Although nothing beats fresh berries for a snack, reach for frozen fruit to make frosty smoothies year-round. Feel free to mix up your berry choices—strawberries and blackberries work just as well. Make sure to use ground flaxseeds rather than whole flaxseeds.

MAKE-AHEAD TIP: Pour the smoothie into a shaker bottle. Store it in the refrigerator until ready to serve. Add ice as desired and shake well before serving.

- 1   cup frozen raspberries
- ¼   cup frozen blueberries
- ½   orange, peeled
- 2   tablespoons vanilla or unflavored protein powder
- 1   tablespoon ground flaxseeds

In a blender or food processor, combine the raspberries, blueberries, orange, protein powder, and flaxseeds. Blend until of desired consistency.

Nutrition Info
Calories: 270
Total Fat: 5 grams
Carbs: 34 grams
Protein: 27 grams
Fiber: 11 grams

Very Berry Smoothie

Serves 1

Feel free to vary the berry with the season for this sweet treat. Nothing in season? Frozen berries work perfectly!

NUTRITION TIP: Blending a whole orange rather than using juice means you get all the fiber and vitamins from the orange, with none of the fillers or sugar that juices sometimes contain.

$^3/_4$ cup fresh or frozen raspberries

$^3/_4$ cup fresh or frozen pitted cherries

$^1/_2$–$^3/_4$ cup fat-free milk, almond milk, or soy milk

1   orange, peeled

2   tablespoons vanilla or unflavored protein powder

In a blender or food processor, combine the raspberries, cherries, milk, orange, and protein powder. Blend until of desired consistency.

Nutrition Info
Calories: 275
Total Fat: 5 grams
Carbs: 42 grams
Protein: 21 grams
Fiber: 10 grams

Stonefruit Smoothie

Serves 1

In most instances, we prefer fresh fruit to frozen. For smoothies, however, frozen fruit adds a refreshing icy texture to the drink.

SHOPPING TIP: If the peaches at your market are mealy, reach for frozen. No apricots? Substitute more peaches.

2   peaches, pit removed and chopped

1   apricot, pit removed and chopped

1   cup fresh or frozen strawberries

6   ounces fat-free plain Greek yogurt

2   tablespoons ground flaxseeds

1   cup small ice cubes or chips

In a blender or food processor, combine the peaches, apricot, strawberries, yogurt, flaxseeds, and ice. Blend until of desired consistency.

Nutrition Info
Calories: 310
Total Fat: 7 grams
Carbs: 46 grams
Protein: 20 grams
Fiber: 11 grams

PB&J Smoothie

Serves 1

Your favorite sandwich flavors can be transformed into a satisfying midday drink.

STORAGE TIP: Got overripe berries or fruit? Don't throw it out—instead freeze it for smoothies. Prep and chop the fruit so it's ready to use; you can just throw it all in the same bag.

2   cups chopped fresh or frozen strawberries

1   frozen banana, chopped

2   teaspoons peanut butter

4   ounces fat-free plain Greek yogurt or fat-free milk

½   cup ice cubes or chips

In a blender or food processor, combine the strawberries, banana, peanut butter, yogurt, and ice. Blend until of desired consistency.

Nutrition Info
Calories: 310
Total Fat: 7 grams
Carbs: 47 grams
Protein: 17 grams
Fiber: 9 grams

Raspberry Lemon Drop Smoothie

Serves 1

Just for fun, garnish your glass with a twist of lemon peel.

SHOPPING TIP: Too busy to juice lemons? Look for real lemon juice in the refrigerator section of your supermarket.

1	cup frozen raspberries
12	raw cashews
3	tablespoons lemon juice
6	ounces fat-free plain Greek yogurt
¾	cup ice chips or cubes
	Twist of lemon peel (optional)

In a blender or food processor, combine the raspberries, cashews, lemon juice, yogurt, ice, and lemon peel, if desired. Blend until of desired consistency.

Nutrition Info
Calories: 274
Total Fat: 9 grams
Carbs: 31 grams
Protein: 21 grams
Fiber: 10 grams

GREEN SMOOTHIES

Sweet Spinach Smoothie

Serves 1

A spinach smoothie is a great way to add leafy greens to your diet. Here, spinach is paired with sweet grapes and pears, creamy yogurt, avocado, and a splash of lime juice. For best flavor, select a ripe pear for this recipe.

STORAGE TIP: Since you are using only part of the avocado, carve out a slice, then tightly wrap the remaining avocado in plastic wrap and refrigerate it until you need it again.

- 2 cups spinach leaves, packed
- 1 ripe pear, peeled, cored and chopped
- 15 green or red grapes
- 6 ounces fat-free plain Greek yogurt
- 2 tablespoons chopped avocado
- 1—2 tablespoons fresh lime juice

In a blender or food processor, combine the spinach, pear, grapes, yogurt, avocado, and lime juice to taste. Blend until of desired consistency.

Nutrition Info
Calories: 315
Total Fat: 7 grams
Carbs: 43 grams
Protein: 25 grams
Fiber: 9 grams

Green Mango Smoothie

Serves 1

Although we feature Swiss chard in this drink, you can always substitute spinach, kale, or any dark leafy green.

TECHNIQUE TIP: Remember to trim the chard before adding it to the blender. The thick woody stems are too tough to include in the smoothie.

- 1½ cups chopped Swiss chard
- 1 cup fresh or frozen mango chunks
- ½ cup fresh or frozen blueberries
- 2 tablespoons unflavored protein powder
- ½ cup ice cubes or chips

In a blender or food processor, combine the Swiss chard, mango, blueberries, protein powder, and ice. Blend until of desired consistency.

Nutrition Info
Calories: 320
Total Fat: 2 grams
Carbs: 64 grams
Protein: 20 grams
Fiber: 9 grams

Kiwi-Strawberry Smoothie

Serves 1

Baby arugula adds a peppery bite to this refreshing drink. These delicate, tiny leaves are a super-flexible ingredient; they're delicious eaten fresh in salads, cooked as a side dish, or swirled into a smoothie.

TECHNIQUE TIP: In order to up the fiber content, include the skin of fruits like apples, peaches, and pears in your smoothies. For this smoothie, you'll need to peel the kiwifruit; the skin is too tough.

2	cups baby arugula
2	kiwifruit, peeled and chopped
5	fresh or frozen strawberries, chopped
1	frozen banana, chopped
2	tablespoons protein powder

In a blender or food processor, combine the arugula, kiwis, strawberries, banana, and protein powder. Blend until of desired consistency.

Nutrition Info
Calories: 300
Total Fat: 3 grams
Carbs: 54 grams
Protein: 21 grams
Fiber: 9 grams

Cool Cucumber-Lime Smoothie

Serves 1

1	small cucumber, peeled and seeded
1	tablespoon fresh lime juice
10	frozen green grapes
6	ounces fat-free Greek yogurt
$\frac{1}{2}$	cup ice cubes or chips
	Fresh mint leaf, for garnish

In a blender or food processor, combine the cucumber, lime juice, grapes, yogurt, and ice. Blend until of desired consistency. Garnish with the mint leaf.

Nutrition Info
Calories: 320
Total Fat: 1 gram
Carbs: 63 grams
Protein: 22 grams
Fiber: 6 grams

Caribbean Kale Smoothie

Serves 1

Coconut extract adds a taste of the tropics to this satisfying drink.

TECHNIQUE TIP: For ease in blending, use crushed ice.

1	cup chopped kale
1	small frozen banana, chopped
1	cup frozen mango chunks
2	tablespoons unflavored protein powder
$\frac{1}{2}$	teaspoon coconut extract
1	cup ice cubes or chips

In a blender or food processor, combine the kale, banana, mango, protein powder, coconut extract, and ice. Blend until of desired consistency.

Nutrition Info
Calories: 310
Total Fat: 2 grams
Carbs: 56 grams
Protein: 26 grams
Fiber: 9 grams

OTHER DELICIOUS SMOOTHIES TO TRY

Maxwell Mocha Smoothie

1	scoop chocolate whey powder
2	teaspoons chia seed powder
1	cup almond milk
1–2	shots espresso (cooled)
1	tablespoon stevia
	Ice

Piña Colada Smoothie

1	orange, peeled
1/3	cup coconut milk
1	scoop whey protein powder
1	banana
1	cup pineapple chunks

Chocolate Smoothie

1	banana
2	tablespoons unsweetened cocoa powder
1	scoop whey protein powder
1	cup almond milk
1	tablespoon stevia (or sweetener of your choice)
5	almonds

7

Learning to Move

All right, now that you've got the eating part down, let's talk about exercise, yet another aspect of weight loss that has gotten completely out of control. Here, too, we desperately need to press the reset button. Most people who want to lose weight fall under two categories. Some don't move enough, and others move too intensely. There's no greater symbol of this ridiculous extreme behavior than the fitness infomercials that flood our airwaves in the wee hours of the night. One of the top-selling fitness programs right now is actually called INSANITY,® which perfectly describes our state of mind as well as the fitness fads we're so impulsively embracing one after the other.

Here's what these programs and the mind-set behind them are doing to us. We're getting injured. We have bad knees, bad posture, excessive soreness. And yet, we can't maintain a trim physique long-term. On the one hand, we're working out so hard, yet we're getting almost NO exercise in our day-to-day lives. How could we possibly take the stairs when our butts are still aching from last week's P90X workout?! Our over-the-top exercise regimens are also supercharging our appetites and causing us to overeat, and overeating makes us fat. It doesn't help that when we work out so hard, we are blasting our bodies with huge amounts of the hormone cortisol, which studies have shown can increase levels of body fat.[1] Study after study has concluded that while moderate exercise has a protective effect on the body, improving general health and longevity, too much exercise can have the opposite effect.[2]

Stop feeling guilty about not going to the gym every morning before work. We have more gyms than any country on earth—and more obese people. And why is that? Leaving aside our poor eating habits for the moment, one big reason is that we're not active enough in the right way.

But wait, you say. Laziness is not my issue. I am a total gym addict. I go every single day after work. Fine, well—what do you do the rest of the time? The fundamental problem here isn't that we're not devoted enough to our burn-500-calories-in-an-hour spin regimen. It's that we've created this completely skewed situation in which we can exercise only at a certain time of day in a certain room in a certain building with a certain piece of equipment.

Our fitness hang-ups are yet another symptom of our efficient-to-a-fault lifestyles. Even if we do work out several times a week, we tend to spend the rest of the time not moving at all. Most of us sit at a desk for 8 hours a day and on a couch for another 8. Those of us who are exercising at all tend to be exercising too intensely and leading inactive lives, and the imbalance is catching up with us.

I have a news flash for you: The manic exercisers so fond of going overboard at the gym are by no means at uniformly healthy body weights, and nor are they particularly satisfied with their physiques. On the contrary, their weights tend to fluctuate regularly and in some cases dramatically for the reasons I've already described: because they're injuring themselves, because they're overeating, and because they're playing havoc with their stress hormones. Oh, and let's not forget that, like the rest of us, they're simply not moving enough in the rest of their lives.

As for the first issue: These hard-core exercisers may well be investing time and sometimes serious money trying to get fit, but if they're eating an extra 1,000 calories a day for every hour they work out, they're ultimately undermining their efforts. To shed pounds, you *must* cut back on calories—but it's very hard to do this when you're running 12 miles before breakfast.

I'm not saying we don't need ANY exercise—not at all. Physical activity is *extremely* important, and our general lack of it is one of the main reasons we're so unhealthy as a culture. Activity improves our quality of life in ways big and small. It makes lifting suitcases and walking up the stairs easier; it relieves stress and improves posture. Regular movement boosts what the World Health Organization calls "healthy life expectancy," and it might even help us sleep.[3] It has a number of these more abstract benefits, like helping to relieve mild to moderate depression.[4] Recent studies have shown that exercise can make cancer treatments more effective.[5] Exercise can help repair the body, as well as help to prevent injuries in the first place.[6]

So yes, exercise is essential. But the big question is how much and what type.

First, we need to learn how to differentiate between "exercise" as we currently understand it—i.e., something that can be done only inside a gym, at a designated time with a designated piece of equipment—and activity. Activity is a submaximal (below maximum) steady state of physical movement, a means of expending energy without forcing us to carve out a separate time from our days. Walking over to the copy machine, getting up to answer the phone, even fidgeting—all count as activity.

Unlike "exercise," physical activity is not scheduled or contrived but rather a naturally occurring part of our everyday lives. And, most important, this type of regular, day-to-day movement does not cause our appetite to spike and induce us to eat more than we otherwise would. One recent study found that people preferred more "high-fat sweet foods" immediately after exercising, thereby diminishing the likelihood of fat loss from the exercise.[7]

The key, then, is not to sweat till you drop, but rather to move constantly around the clock. Moreover, it's time to dispel one of the greatest myths around sweating: It doesn't equal burning fat! If you're sitting in a chair on a hot day and you sweat, you're not burning fat.

Instead of sending an e-mail to your colleague 10 cubicles away, walk over to ask the question in person. Instead of drinking your morning coffee in bed, throw on some sweatpants and drink it while strolling around the block. The list of possibilities goes on and on. Get up from your desk every 20 minutes. Buy a hands-free headset for your phone, and the next time you're on a call, take it while pacing your office or tidying the house. Don't just hunch over in your chair or stretch out on the couch. Leave your phone across the room so that you have to get up every time it beeps. Don't yell for someone else to answer the door when the UPS guy comes calling—get up and answer it yourself. When your favorite writer has a new book out, download an audio version of it and listen to it while walking to work instead of while lying in bed.

I promise you, all these little efforts will pay big dividends. Everything counts. Walking to the bathroom, going to the ATM on foot—all of these movements contribute to your overall well-being. Even the smallest movements—what are known as incidental physical activities—can make a big difference in your overall cardiorespiratory fitness, a recent study found.[8] Another study found that sedentary overweight or obese middle-aged women can vastly improve their health with as little as 10 minutes of exercise a day—that's time well spent![9]

I guarantee that a person who's moderately active all day long—who always takes the stairs, who takes a lap around the office every 20 minutes—will be much healthier than someone who has a completely sedentary lifestyle but works out hard at a few pre-planned intervals several times a week.

This regular motion will have another side effect as well: It will keep you occupied, which is a good thing. Too often, overeating is a direct result of boredom and the desire for distraction, both of which are by-products of our all-too-sedentary lives. So whatever you do, get up and MOVE—especially while you're still getting the hang of this new system, when you're most likely to be tempted to snack for no reason.

How to Move in Phase I

I've said it before and I'll say it again: It's important to be physically active as long as you don't overdo it. It doesn't have to be vigorous or backbreaking. It just has to be regular physical activity.

That's why, for the duration of Phase I, we'll keep it super simple on the exercise front, sticking to one and only one activity: walking. Walking is absolutely crucial to our continued good health, and it's a key determinant of countries with long life spans. One study found that women who walked at a moderate pace for as little as an hour a week significantly cut their risk of heart disease.[10] Regular walking has also been shown to reduce blood pressure, lower the risk of diabetes and strokes, and increase lung capacity.

A collaborative study involving 14 researchers from the United States, Australia, Canada, France, and Sweden established preliminary guidelines for how many steps per day people should take for weight control, and the number they've hit upon is 10,000. Many Americans barely walk 3,000 steps most days—is it any wonder we're so fat and unhealthy?[11] A recent study found that the morbidly obese were sedentary for more than 99 percent of the day and, on average, walked fewer than 2,500 steps per day.

So 10,000 steps a day is the magic number here, a goal you'll be tracking with the help of a pedometer, a step-counting device that you can easily keep in your pocket. Ten thousand steps is about 4 miles, which can sound like a pretty daunting number, but I promise you it's not; after all, we're counting every step you take from the minute you get up in the morning until the minute you go to bed.

For the first 15 days of this plan, you will carry your pedometer

Picking Out the
Perfect Pedometer

Pedometers can have an impressive impact on how much you walk: Studies have shown that wearing a pedometer can help increase people's awareness of their physical movements—and then, with any luck, increase their actual movements. A Stanford University study found that people who wore pedometers increased their physical activity by 27 percent, or about 2,000 steps (1 mile) every day. They also lowered their body mass index (BMI).

Pedometers are extremely inexpensive; a basic model can cost as little as $10. They're also versatile devices. You can toss one in your pocket or strap one to your hip; you can even buy a pedometer that looks exactly like a digital watch. The possibilities are endless. One cool little gadget, the Fitbit, is small enough to be clipped onto a bra strap and tabulates how much you sleep in addition to how much you move. We also love the simplicity of the New Balance Slim.

Easy Ways to **Hit 10,000**

- First thing in the morning, walk around the block.
- Leave the car at home and take the bus to work. Or, if public transportation isn't convenient, start a carpool with a neighbor and walk to that neighbor's house on foot. Get in the habit of parking in the most inconvenient, distant spot in the lot.
- Skip the escalator or elevator and take the stairs instead.
- At airports, skip the moving walkways and hoof it to the gate without technological assistance.
- Walk up and down every single aisle of the grocery store every single time you go shopping.

everywhere you go. You might be surprised by how much (or how little) you walk in an average day.

In the beginning, you might have to plot out exactly how to achieve this baseline goal of 10,000 steps. And as with any life modification, there will be challenging moments, though I'd wager that these will be more psychological than physical. Getting to 10,000 steps can be as simple as taking a loop around the block before each meal or snack, or playing a game of pickup basketball for 20 minutes (which is how long it took me to hit 10,000 steps when I played last week). And whatever you do, make sure you take the stairs whenever possible.

I'm not saying that you can't *ever* use a treadmill at the gym—not at all. I'm saying that hitting the treadmill shouldn't be the be-all and end-all of your daily physical activity. Gym-going is a type of compensation for the exercise you're not getting in the rest of your life, meaning if it's 9 p.m. and you've managed to walk only 2,000 steps from the moment you woke up, then you need to either take a walk outside or spend a half hour on the treadmill. But these measures should be the exception, not the norm.

Remember, we are trying to avoid supercharging your appetite in these first few days. High-intensity bouts of exercise will not be assisting your efforts here. Instead, concentrate on reaching that 10,000-step mark before bedtime every night.

PHASE I SAMPLE SCHEDULE

6:30 a.m.	Wake up
6:45 a.m.	After a shower, take your morning cup of coffee and walk around the block: 1,500 steps.
7:15 a.m.	Breakfast: white smoothie
7:45 a.m.	Walk to the bus, or if you drive to work, make another quick loop around the block before getting into the car: 1,500 steps.
8:15 a.m.	Once at work, take the stairs, or arrive a little early so that you can take a quick walk to the newsstand a block away: 2,000 steps.
10:30 a.m.	Morning snack: 1 large Bosc pear + 2 slices of turkey. Walk downstairs and enjoy it on a bench outside: 1,000 steps.
1:00–1:15 p.m.	Lunch: red smoothie
1:15–2:00 p.m.	Spend the rest of your lunch break running errands on foot (picking up your dry cleaning, stopping by the coffee shop for another coffee). Or just catch up with your mom by telephone while you stroll through the neighborhood: 3,000 steps.
4:15 p.m.	Afternoon snack: 4 slices Finn Crisp crackers + 2 slices fat-free cheese. Now head down to a nearby coffee shop for an iced green tea to get you through those last few hours of work.
6:45 p.m.	Stop off at the grocery store on your way home. Remember to park in the most inconvenient spot in the lot, and be sure to walk every aisle: 1,500 steps. Congrats: You've hit your 10,000-step mark!
7:15 p.m.	Snack: green smoothie

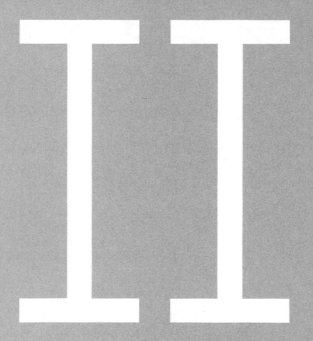

PHASE II

8

Making the Transition

Phase II: What You'll Be Doing

You will be eating five times a day: two smoothies, two snacks, and one single-dish meal. You will be walking a minimum of 10,000 steps and beginning a simple circuit of resistance training 3 days a week (or on Days 6, 8, and 10 of the plan).

What You'll Need

- A blender
- A pedometer
- A shopping list

You've done it! You've made it through the first, and surely the hardest, 5 days of the plan. I'd wager that you're looking and feeling pretty good right about now. How many pounds have you lost? Three? Five? Even more?

In any event, the dramatic results you've experienced in the last 5 days have surely been great motivation to continue on with the Body Reset. I promise you it only gets easier at every phase as you gradually ease your way back into the "real world."

The big dietary change in Phase II is that you'll now be replacing one of your three daily smoothies with a satisfying single-dish meal. I don't mind which meal you replace—it really depends on your schedule and your eating habits.

Ask yourself when you're most vulnerable to pigging out and try to keep that meal as a smoothie. For me, dinner is the toughest time to keep my discipline intact, so that's the best time for me to have a smoothie. But efficiency is also a factor—when are you most crunched for time? If your morning routine is frenzied, then maybe it makes the most sense to have a smoothie then, when you don't have time to prepare even the simplest meal. If it's quicker for you to bring your red smoothie to lunch in a thermos, then by all means do that, and have your S-meal at home with your family at night. If you like the ritual of slowing down and eating a meal with a plate and fork in the little park outside your office building, then bring one of the S-meals with you.

You can work out the details according to your own preferences and time constraints. There just has to be a method to the madness, so figure out what your method is.

Restoring a Passion for Eating

Sooner or later (preferably sooner), after a jump start like Phase I of this plan, we have to make the transition back to single-dish meals. Solid meals take longer to consume than even the most fiber-packed smoothies, and our bodies generally absorb them more slowly, both of which are good for weight loss. And there's a social aspect to eating that most diets overlook—and because they overlook it, those diets tend not to be sustainable. We are social creatures, and we can go only so long drinking every meal on our own. The smoothie is absolutely critical for the success of the kick start: It is the most efficient, nutrient-packed way to shed pounds fast without devoting your entire day to obsessing about weight loss.

So while there is only so much variety you can get from a blender, and variety—of texture, flavor, and color—it's also important to include other aspects of eating. Solid foods can give you a satisfying variety that smoothies cannot. Solid foods also take longer to digest, and sitting down to eat them is your chance to breathe and recharge. When you eat solid foods, your mouth acts as the blender, and you need to take time to ensure that it does its work properly.

Digestion, after all, starts in your mouth, both in its mechanical aspects, which set off a whole cascade of digestive processes in your stomach, and in the enzymes released by your saliva. So when you slow down to chew every bite carefully, you'll increase the amount of nutrients absorbed into your body.

So let's start to make the transition back to solid foods. Of course, whenever you get too busy or hectic or feel the need to reset your habits again (or shed more weight in a hurry), you can always turn back to the three-smoothies-a-day tool, but I don't really think it's realistic to live primarily off smoothies for the rest of your life. One to two smoothies a day, however, *is* sustainable, so that's what you'll transition to in Phase III and beyond.

Restoring a passion for eating is central to the long-term success of this plan. Yes, we all lead fast-paced lives and seldom come up for air. But when we pay too little attention to what we're putting into our mouths, we keep on eating and eating regardless of whether we're still hungry or even whether we like the food! I want you to reclaim not only a healthy lifestyle, but the enjoyment of the ritual of eating—gathering around the table with friends and loved ones, savoring every morsel of both food and conversation.

What You'll Be Learning: Basic Food Prep

The first thing I want to emphasize is that my recipes are EASY, so don't feel overwhelmed. The time commitment involved in making these meals will be 5 minutes or less, I promise. You *can* (and will!) prepare simple, delicious, and nourishing meals in a snap.

Taking control of your body (and what goes in it) does call for a measure of self-reliance in the kitchen, but that doesn't mean that cooking has to be a headache—on the contrary. These recipes will show you exactly how easy it can be to make great food.

To show you just how simple cooking can be, we'll be starting with super-easy one-dish meals like stir-fries and soups that adhere to the basic principles of the Body Reset, meaning they all contain a great balance of proteins, fiber, and healthy fats, and they all take under 5 minutes to prepare. Their nutritional profile—calorie count and fiber and protein content—is roughly equivalent to that of the smoothies; the main difference is that we consume them with a knife and fork instead of a straw.

Mastering Basic
Meal Preparation

Learning to prepare your own meals can fundamentally change the way you eat, and the Body Reset meals are the perfect springboard for cooks of all experience levels, from gourmet chefs to total kitchen-phobes. Studies show that people who prepare meals at home feel more emotionally rewarded after eating them. When you're preparing your own food, you also know exactly what's in every meal, which is not usually true of meals you order at restaurants or pick up in convenient little boxes in the freezer section of the supermarket. It should come as no surprise that food prepared at home tends to have a much lower calorie count than food ordered in a restaurant. An average restaurant meal contains between 1,000 and 2,000 calories, or between 50 percent and 100 percent of the total calories you should consume daily. By following *The Body Reset Diet,* you won't be frequenting restaurants as often as the average American, who eats out at least five meals weekly. Self-reliance in the kitchen and a tendency to eat more at home will yield big savings—in both the wallet and the waistline—over the years.

The key to these meals is **SIMPLICITY**, which is why I call them **S-meals**. S stands for both **Simple** and **Single dish**, and also for the actual type of dishes:

- Salads
- Sandwiches
- Soups
- Stir-fries
- Scrambles

Simple = No Excuses. These meals are simple in terms of time, accessibility of ingredients, and preparation method—and simply delicious!

On page 183, I'll give you many options for each of these recipes. You can have Sweet Potato Hash with Chives (page 189) on Day 6, and try out the Southwestern Tuna Tortilla Wrap (page 198) on Day 7. There's something for everyone, and I promise that no matter how inexperienced you are in the kitchen, you *will* be able to make these meals in no time at all—and feel that much more satisfied with the food (and yourself) for having done it on your own.

Later, as you move into the rest of your life phase, I encourage you to pick up some of my previous books to experiment with more delicious simple recipes. Those recipes are also incredibly filling, and a cinch to prepare no matter what your time constraints. But for now, let's stick to the one-dish meals, like the amazing Tuscan White Bean and Kale Bruschetta (page 220) and the mouthwatering Dijon Lentil Salad with Baby Spinach (page 212), which are truly as **Simple** as it gets!

Planning Ahead

Just as in Phase I, to succeed in Phase II you need to do some advance planning. Before you go to bed, think about what you'll eat the next day. Although this plan allows you to be flexible about what you eat, I do want you to continue alternating the smoothies in pretty much the same order, even as you go down to two a day. Over the years, I've found that establishing a routine helps you succeed in planning ahead to prepare meals. Obviously, the choices you make will really depend on your mood, and when you'll be in your kitchen and when you'll be on the move, and what you ate the day before and what you happen to have in your pantry.

The following chart is by no means a hard-and-fast template. It's merely an attempt to show you how you can alternate your meals and smoothies for maximum flexibility. If you strongly prefer the white to the red smoothie, then you can have the white smoothie more often, but please don't exclude one type entirely. These smoothies were designed to give you the proper balance of nutrients when eaten in alternation. Try to rotate them.

The same goes for the S-meals. If it's the sweltering middle of summer, I totally understand that you won't be eating as many hot soups, but that doesn't mean you have to eat the exact same sandwich every single day. The success of a diet depends on variety, so try to eat as many different dishes as you can, especially early on when you're still figuring out what works for you.

PHASE II

	Day 6	Day 7	Day 8	Day 9	Day 10
Breakfast	White smoothie	Green smoothie	Red smoothie	S-meal	Green smoothie
Snack 1	Snack	Snack	Snack	Snack	Snack
Lunch	Red smoothie	S-meal	Green smoothie	White smoothie	S-meal
Snack 2	Snack	Snack	Snack	Snack	Snack
Dinner	S-meal	White smoothie	S-meal	Red smoothie	White smoothie

Some Preliminary Tips for Transitioning Back to Solid Meals

- Try to eat your solid meals while sitting down (and no, driving doesn't count). Put down your phone, turn off the TV, and try to focus on what you're eating for the few minutes that you have. Enjoy your meals and you won't find yourself mindlessly snacking quite so often.

- Plot out your mealtimes well in advance. Don't get yourself in a situation where you're so ravenously hungry that you eat everything in sight.

- Chew your food slowly and deliberately.

- When you have eaten three-quarters of the food on your plate, wait several minutes and see if you're still hungry or if you can save that portion for leftovers.

Easing into Resistance Training

Now that your body has adapted to the smoothies and you'll be incorporating one solid S-meal into your daily diet, you're ready to start a little resistance training in addition to walking your usual 10,000 steps a day. (Meeting that goal has gotten pretty easy already, hasn't it? Ever glance down at your pedometer and feel surprised by how many steps you've walked without even trying?)

Resistance training—a type of strength training defined by resistance to a specific force of opposition—is an essential component of long-term good health. Resistance training can include everything from calisthenics (using your own body weight) to free weights. Pilates and yoga also fall into this category, though they are both submaximal forms of resistance training, meaning they have a good deal of value but aren't quite intense enough to create the dramatically sculpted body we're trying to achieve.

According to the Centers for Disease Control, resistance training can be a powerful weapon against a wide range of maladies, from obesity and diabetes to back pain and arthritis. And it's long been known that weight-bearing activity can improve muscle and bone density and therefore prevent osteoporosis.[1] Resistance training is our very best defense against chronic pain, and it can even fight depression. It's particularly important as we get older, helping to counteract muscle atrophy and maintain mobility.[2]

While resistance training is not, strictly speaking, about burning calories—the point is more to sculpt your body and rev your resting metabolism to ensure that you're burning calories even when you sleep—its benefits are even more powerful for people trying to lose weight. Resistance training twice a week has been shown to improve resting metabolism and to reduce insulin resistance, body fat, and high blood pressure.[3] It's also the best way to tone and tighten your body; no diet, however healthy, can do this for you. But how much is enough? How can we make strengthening our bodies a sustainable daily activity for the rest of our lives?

As always, less is more. In spite of what you see at the gym or read in magazines, you do NOT have to go overboard. A recent study concluded that heavy weights aren't necessary for improving body strength: You can build the same amount of strength from lifting lighter weights more times as from killing yourself by lifting heavier weights a few

No Excuses!

The Body Reset resistance program could not be easier.
   It doesn't require any equipment.
   It takes less than 5 minutes from start to finish.
   It consists of incredibly simple moves,

times.[4] You don't have to push your muscles to their limit (and thereby increase your risk of injury) to get the strongest body of your life. What matters more is being consistent, and doing enough sets to tire out your muscles.

Together with your new diet, the Body Reset circuits I've designed are THE shortest, simplest path to the strong, sexy body you've always wanted. The four exercises you'll do in Phase II are extremely easy to perform and take only 5 minutes out of your busy schedule, 3 days a week. *You don't even need any equipment*—no dumbbells, no fancy gym machines—to see amazing results. (If you choose the more advanced exercises, you have the option of including a couple of dumbbells and a stability ball, but the program is otherwise equipment free.) The weight of your body is sufficient to get you in great shape in no time. You also don't need to do a million sets to start feeling serious, and seriously exciting, changes in your body. Often doing 1 set can be just as effective, which is why we're starting you off with a single set.

Whatever your current fitness level, doing these circuits is a small investment with huge rewards. These exercises will make ALL the difference to the health of your body.

Circuit A

In Phase II, you'll be doing **Circuit A** 3 days a week. This circuit consists of four simple exercises designed to train the **posterior muscles** of your body. These are the muscles attached to the back of your body.

The main posterior muscles we'll be working include:

- Your upper back (rhomboids)
- The back of your arms (triceps)
- Your lower back (spinal erectors)
- The back of your thighs (hamstrings and glutes)

Training posterior muscles is crucially important because over time, our sedentary lifestyles have given rise to poor posture that can lead to major injuries. Every aspect of our daily lives causes us to hunch forward: We spend all day leaning into our computers, our phones, the steering wheel. Women in particular, who are often self-conscious about sticking out their chests, tend to walk hunched forward.

Our exercise habits aren't helping matters much, either. We do far too many crunches, chest flys, and biceps curls—exercises that work our already-overused anterior, or front, muscles. By doing more posterior than anterior work, we are undoing all the damage our lifestyles have done to our bodies over time. Posterior muscles help correct our imbalances and address postural issues, but they can also make our arms and our midsections—the distance between our breastbone and belly button—look longer and leaner, giving us a natural chest lift. (This benefits both women *and* men—nobody wants flabby-looking pectorals!) Posterior exercises also drastically tone the back of your legs where your thighs meet your butt, and *everybody* wants that.

Depending on your fitness level going into the Body Reset, you can modify the exercises as explained on the next few pages.

How Do I Know
If I'm a Beginner?

I've custom-designed these exercises for three different fitness levels: beginner, intermediate, and advanced. Here's how to figure out where you fall on the spectrum.

You're a beginner if you're currently sedentary, do not exercise regularly, and have done little or no resistance training in the past.

You're intermediate if you've done some resistance training in the past and are somewhat active (i.e., you work out at least twice a week).

You're advanced if you're very familiar with resistance training and currently do some form of resistance training 2 or 3 days a week.

How Many?

Beginners: Do 20 repetitions of each exercise; do one circuit.

Intermediate: Do 20 repetitions of each exercise; do two circuits.

Advanced: Do 20 repetitions of each exercise; do three circuits.

If you're starting as a beginner, you will add an extra circuit every month, until you are up to three circuits. Once you have been doing three circuits for several months, you can progress to the intermediate and then the advanced movements. At the same time, you'll be adjusting the movements you're doing as your body gets stronger.

This progression—adding more repetitions and different variations as you acclimate to the exercises—is extremely important. For your body to progress, your fitness program must progress as well.

That's why I've built two different types of progression into this program: first, via the actual level of difficulty of the exercise (I offer modifications for beginner, intermediate, and advanced levels); and second, via the number of repetitions and sets of the exercise. You'll start in Phase I doing no resistance exercise just walking, then proceed to doing circuits three and then five times a week. As your strength builds, you will add more complicated variations and increase the number of sets you do. No matter which phase you're in, you'll always be walking 10,000 steps a day.

It's also important to understand that the key to resistance training is not the calories you'll burn while doing it, but the residual increase in your metabolism that results from doing the exercises. The more toned our bodies, the more efficient our resting metabolism, and the more calories we burn—even while we're sleeping. In addition to walking 10,000 steps a day, you're continually burning fat *while* you're moving, but by doing these resistance exercises, you're training your body to burn fat *after* you're done moving.

How Often?

In Phase II, you will do Circuit A on 3 days: Days 6, 8, and 10 (and 3 nonconsecutive days a week thereafter).

The Exercises

EXERCISE #1: REVERSE FLY

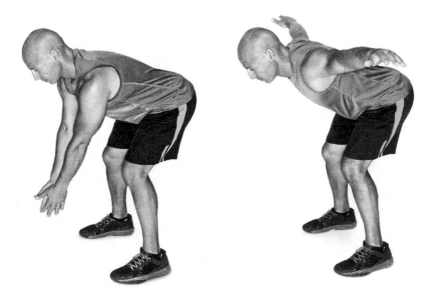

Works: Upper back and shoulders

How to: Stand with your feet shoulder-width apart. Stick your butt out and lean forward until your upper torso is parallel to the floor. Raise your hands out at your sides. (Imagine you are flying away—think of your arms as long wings.) Stop when your arms are parallel to the floor, then slowly lower your arms back down toward your sides. Keep a slight bend in your elbows throughout the exercise and squeeze your shoulder blades together at the top of the movement.

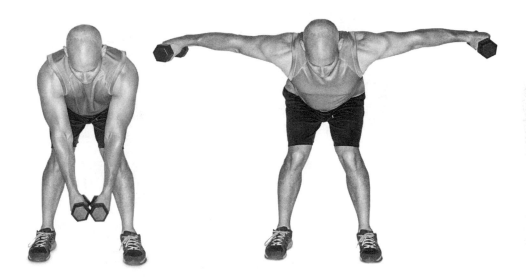

Intermediate: Add 16-ounce water bottles, one in each hand, first filled a quarter of the way with water, then halfway, then all the way, according to your strength level.

Advanced *(shown above)*: Replace the water bottles with light dumbbells.

EXERCISE #2: TRICEPS DIP OR LYING TRICEPS EXTENSION

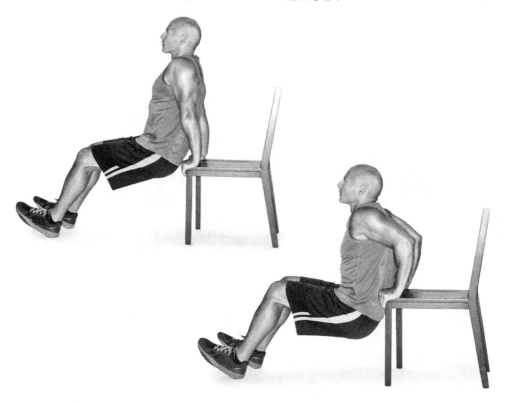

Works: Triceps primarily, but also shoulders and chest

How to: Begin seated on a bench or chair. Put the heels of your hands on the edge of the chair, slide your butt forward, and place your heels about hip-width apart on the floor. Slowly bending your elbows, lower your lower body 6 to 10 inches. Drive through the heels of your palm and contract your triceps. Now press your arms back up until they are straight. Repeat.

Intermediate: Extend your legs farther away from you. They can even be straight. The farther your feet are from your body, the more difficult the exercise.

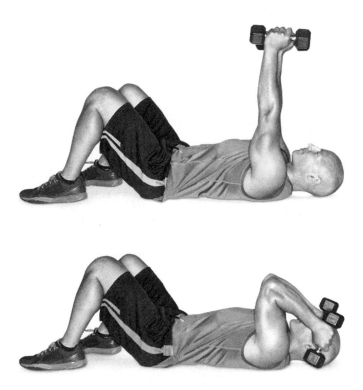

Advanced/Lying Triceps Extension *(shown above)*: Lie on your back with your arms extended straight up toward the ceiling, your palms facing each other, and a dumbbell or water bottle in each hand. Hinging at your elbows, lower the weights down between your shoulders and ears, then extend them toward the ceiling and return to the starting position.

EXERCISE #3: SUPERMAN

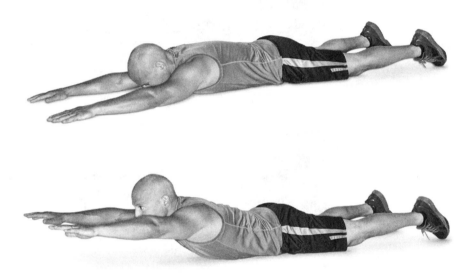

Works: Lower back and butt

How to: Lie facedown on the floor with your arms and legs fully extended. From this position, lift your arms toward the ceiling, as if you were flying. Lower back down and keep repeating.

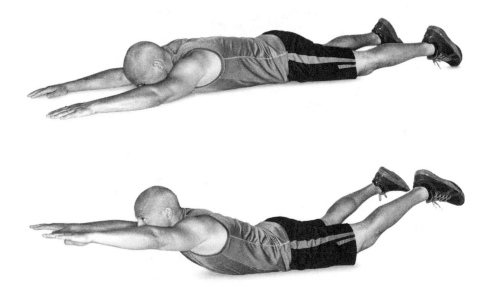

Intermediate: Add your lower body, lifting your legs at the same time as your arms so that your body looks like the letter X from above. Tap the floor with your hands and feet between reps.

Advanced: Don't let your feet or hands touch the floor; keep them moving at all times.

EXERCISE #4: PRONE HAMSTRING CURL OR BALL HAMSTRING CURL

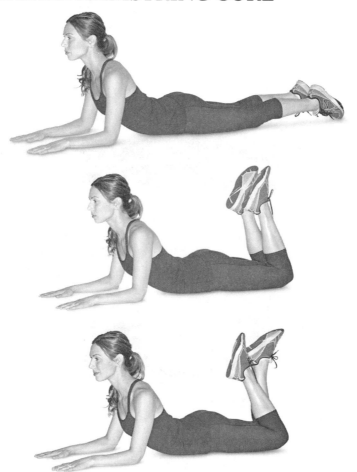

Works: Hamstrings

How to: Lie on your stomach, propped up on your forearms, with your hips down and your back as flat as possible. With your legs relaxed, bring your feet toward your butt.

Intermediate: Lie on your stomach, propped up on your forearms. Rest the laces of your right shoe on top of your left heel. *(See bottom photo.)* Repeat the exercise using your left hamstring, with your right leg working as dead weight. Do all the reps on your left leg, then repeat with your left shoe on top of your right heel.

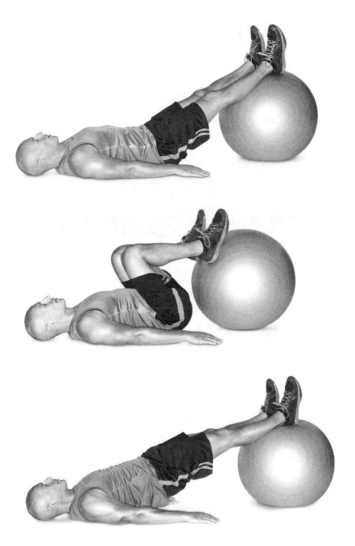

Advanced Ball Hamstring Curl: If you're this advanced, you should invest in a stability ball. (You can buy one at any sporting goods store. The box will indicate, based on your height, which size you should use. Sizes vary from 45 to 85 centimeters; most people will probably use a 55-centimeter ball.) Lying on your back, put your heels up on the ball and lift your hips up off the floor. Keep your hips as high as you can manage. Bending at the knees, roll the ball in toward your butt and then back away from you.

What Else You'll Be Doing

Don't forget to keep walking! In Phase II, you'll continue to meet your goal of 10,000 steps every single day, so remember that pedometer and get moving.

Here's a chart breaking down your movements over the course of Phase II.

Day 6	Day 7	Day 8	Day 9	Day 10
10,000 steps	10,000 steps	10,000 steps	10,000 steps	10,000 steps
Circuit A	—	Circuit A	—	Circuit A

Phase II: Summary

In Phase II, between Days 6 and 10 of the Body Reset, you'll have two smoothies, two C-snacks, and one S-meal a day. You'll be doing one short circuit of weight training on alternate days while continuing to walk 10,000 steps every day.

PHASE

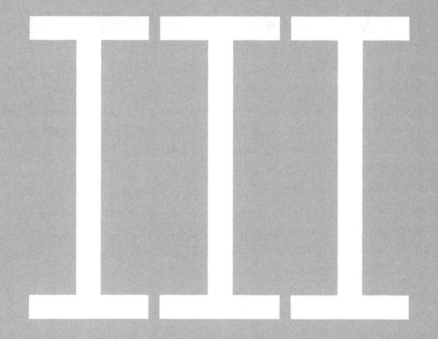

10

Setting the Stage

Phase III: What You'll Be Doing

You will be eating five times a day: one smoothie, two snacks, and two solid meals. You will be walking a minimum of 10,000 steps a day and adding a second resistance circuit on alternate days. You'll still be doing resistance training just 5 minutes a day, but now you'll be doing it 5 days a week instead of just 3.

What You'll Need

- A blender
- A pedometer
- A shopping list

Phase III, which takes place between Days 11 and 15, is your launch-pad to the rest of your life. The eating schedule that you will follow closely resembles—in slightly stricter form—the one you'll adopt once your 15-day reset is complete, meaning you will ultimately enjoy one smoothie a day. You will continue to have two C-snacks daily, but you will also now have the option of two regular S-meals, choosing from the many great salad, sandwich, and scramble recipes I provide in this book.

You will also increase the amount of resistance training you'll be doing, but don't worry—it's nothing too daunting, still just 5 minutes a day, 5 days a week.

Controlling Your Portion Sizes

As you ready yourself to return to the "real world" of eating, you'll need to start thinking not only about WHAT you eat, but HOW MUCH you eat. You can eat the most nutritious ingredients in the world, but if you eat too many of them, you're still going to gain weight. It really is as simple as that.

If, on the other hand, you limit the size of your portions, you can eat pretty much whatever you want (within reason, of course). That's the primary reason the French, whose cuisine is among the richest in the world, are so much thinner than we are: They know that moderation is the key to success in eating.

A good deal of overeating is behavioral, related more to habit than real need. One study found that children as young as 3 years old eat more food if more food is placed in front of them, and the same holds true as we get older: The more food we're served, the more food we eat.[1] On the other hand, if we make an effort to limit our portion sizes, we will eat less food. A study found that people even feed their dogs more depending on the size of the bowl and scoop they use![2] The dogs fed with the largest scoops and bowls weighed more than those fed with regular-size scoops and bowls.

The same holds true for human behavior: It's no surprise that as the size of our dishware has increased in recent decades, so, too, has the size of our jeans.[3] In a recent experiment, participants were given either 34- or 17-ounce bowls and either 2- or 3-ounce serving spoons and told to serve themselves ice cream. The ones with the bigger bowls took 31 percent more ice cream, and the ones with the bigger spoons took 14.5 percent more.[4] Those given both the larger bowls *and* the larger spoons took a whopping 56.8 percent more.

Start paying closer attention to serving sizes, and be mindful of everything you put in your mouth. Though obviously superior to almost any food out there, even certain good-for-you fruits can cause weight gain if eaten in massive enough quantities.[5] Always pay attention to quantity, and know when to say when.

Here are some great tips you can use to control portions.

- Fill up on green salads and soup before the main course. (But avoid full fat dressings and bacon bits!)
- Choose smaller plates so that your eyes don't trick you into eating more food than you need. A reasonable portion of food will be dwarfed by a gigantic dinner plate, so consider eating off smaller side plates.

- Pack your snacks in advance to limit how many you eat. If you have a single-serving bag of soy nuts with you, you will eat only that small bag. If, however, you bring a large package, you are *much* likelier to go overboard and exceed the ½-cup portion.

- Don't eat in front of the TV or computer—there is no better way to lose track of what you're eating (and therefore to eat much more of it than you need) than to eat when you're not paying attention.

- Don't eat buffet-style (except when it comes to salads and fruits). Remember—the more food that's in front of you, the more you're likely to eat. It's easier to avoid having seconds if you have to cross the room to refill your plate.

Planning Ahead

As you continue the transition away from the reset part of the Body Reset, it's more important than ever to figure out when exactly you're going to eat. Is it simplest for you to have your daily smoothie first thing in the morning, when you're trying to do 10 things at once before rushing out the door to work? Then by all means do that. Is it too much trouble to pack a sandwich to take to work and easier to have eggs at home and pack a smoothie to go? Then try that instead.

Again, as long as you plan your mealtimes in advance and try to get as wide a variety of Body Reset foods into your days as possible, you can alternate the foods according to your taste and your schedule. The following chart shows you how easy it is to organize your meals in Phase III.

PHASE III

	Day 11	Day 12	Day 13	Day 14	Day 15
Break-fast	White smoothie	Italian Flag Breakfast Pizza (page 184)	Green smoothie	Herbed Cream Cheese Scramble (page 188)	Red smoothie
Snack 1	Snack	Snack	Snack	Snack	Snack
Lunch	Coconut Chicken Curry (page 221)	Red smoothie	Southwestern Tuna Tortilla Wrap (page 198)	Easy Niçoise Salad (page 215)	Tzatziki Chicken Flatbread (page 200)
Snack 2	Snack	Snack	Snack	Snack	Snack
Dinner	Sunset Squash Soup (page 205)	Sweet Potato Hash with Chives (page 189)	Winter's Day Beef with Barley Soup (page 206)	White smoothie	Grilled Steak and Baby Spin- ach Salad (page 211)

CHAPTER

Increasing the Resistance

The resistance-training component of Phase III is just an extended version of the easy, at-home exercises you've gotten in the swing of doing during Days 6 through 10. It still takes only 5 minutes a day, only this time you'll be alternating between 2 sets of exercises 5 days a week.

The Phase III program consists of **Circuit A**, which you mastered in Phase II, to work all the posterior muscles of your body, and **Circuit B**, which works all the anterior muscles, or the muscles at the front of your body.

The main anterior muscles we'll be working include:

- Your chest (pectorals)

- Your sides (obliques)

- The front of your thighs (quads)

- The front of your midsection (rectus abs)

You'll do Circuit A (see page 120 for descriptions and demonstrations of exercises) on Days 11, 13, and 15, and Circuit B on Days 12 and 14.

Notice how you end up doing three Circuit A routines and only two Circuit B routines per week? That's no accident: It's our way of correcting the muscle imbalances that have built up in our bodies over time. By consistently favoring the anterior over the posterior muscles, we are giving the underused muscles on the backs of our bodies a chance to catch up with our overburdened fronts. That's also why we're doing a plank, instead of a crunch which strengthens the front of our bodies without putting strain on our backs. It's important to work both the anterior and posterior muscles to maintain a straight, strong posture. It's not only good for our bodies but it helps us look great in our clothes, too!

Circuit B

Again, in Phase III, you'll be doing **Circuit A** three times and **Circuit B** twice. Depending on your fitness level going into the Body Reset, you can again modify the exercises as described.

How Many?

Beginners: Do 20 repetitions of each exercise; do one circuit.

Intermediate: Do 20 repetitions of each exercise; do two circuits.

Advanced: Do 20 repetitions of each exercise; do three circuits.

How Often?

In Phase III, you will do Circuit A three times—on Days 11, 13, and 15—and Circuit B twice—on Days 12 and 14.

The Exercises

EXERCISE #1: SQUAT OR SKATER LUNGE

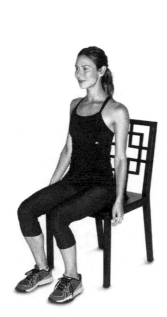
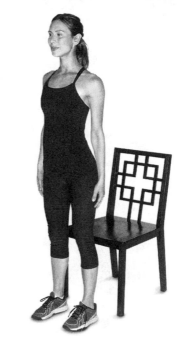

Works: Lower body (glutes, quads, hamstrings)

How to: As you squat and lunge, keep your weight on the arches of your feet and try not to roll onto your toes. Keep looking up the whole time and never lower your butt past your knees. Your thighs should end parallel to the floor.

Intermediate _(shown at right)_: Use a lower seat and continue to sit onto it as before. If you'd like to make it even more difficult, hug a watermelon or add a set of light dumbbells.

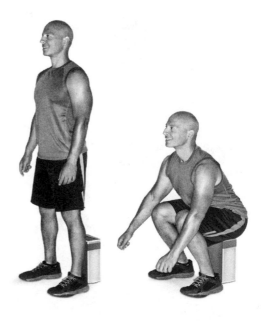

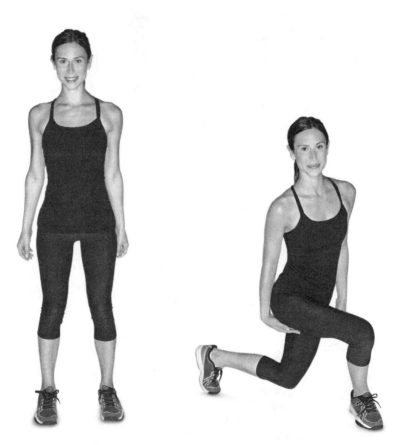

Advanced: Now you're ready for the **Skater Lunge.** Stand with your feet shoulder-width apart. With your right leg, step back and across your body, dropping your right knee behind your left heel. Then return to the beginning stance and do the opposite—step your left leg back and across your body, dropping your left knee behind your right heel. Keep alternating legs, bending one knee to the opposite heel.

EXERCISE #2: MODIFIED PUSHUP

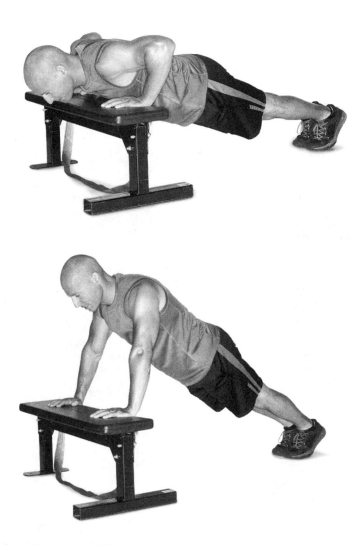

Works: Chest, Shoulders, Triceps

How to: Lean against a bench or countertop. Keep your body rigid and in a straight line. Line up your hands right above your collarbone and nipple line. Bend your elbows and slowly lower your body toward whatever surface you're using. Extend your elbows and repeat.

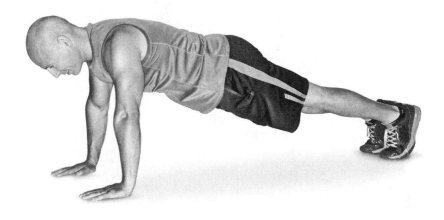

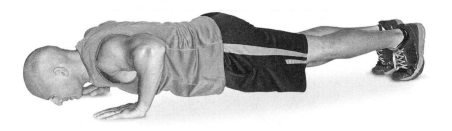

Intermediate: Perform this exercise on the floor with your knees bent and touching the floor and your ankles crossed behind you.

Advanced _(shown above)_: Do a full pushup, with your knees off the floor and your entire body raised.

EXERCISE #3: STANDING SIDE BEND

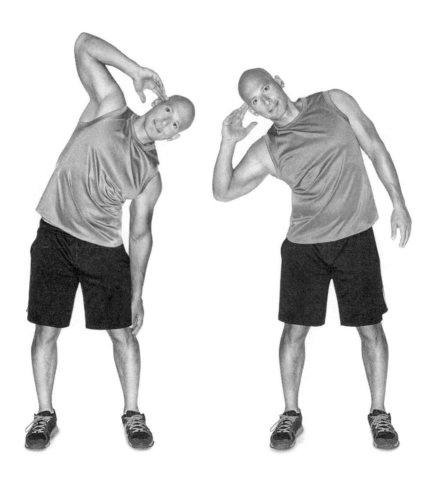

Works: External and internal obliques (aka "love handles")

How to: Stand with your feet shoulder–width apart, with your right index finger and middle finger behind your right ear and your left arm straight against your side. Gently lean your upper body to the right. Repeat in the opposite direction.

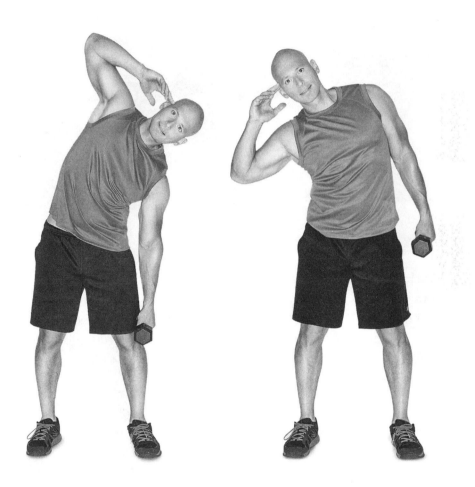

Intermediate/Advanced: Do the exercise with weights—a grocery bag full of canned food, a jug of water, or a dumbbell—in your straight arm.

EXERCISE #4: PLANK

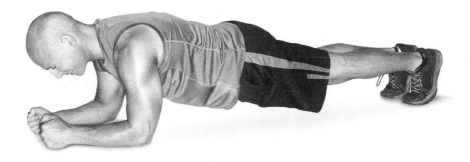

Works: Rectus abdominals (front of your core)

How to: With your elbows bent, rest your forearms on the edge of your bed, or the arm rest of a couch, and extend your legs back so your feet are on the ground and there is a straight line from your heels to your shoulders. Contract your midsection and form a rigid plank with your body.

Intermediate *(shown at left)*: Now perform the same exercise on the floor. Rest your forearms on the floor but allow your hips to be slightly above the plane of your body.

Advanced: Perform the same exercise but make sure your hips are in a straight line with your shoulders and heels.

What Else You'll Be Doing

Meeting your goal of 10,000 daily steps should be second nature by now, allowing you to focus on the expanded resistance training.

Here's a chart to break down your movements over the course of Phase III.

Day 11	Day 12	Day 13	Day 14	Day 15
10,000 steps	10,000 steps	10,000 steps	10,000 steps	10,000 steps
Circuit A	Circuit B	Circuit A	Circuit B	Circuit A

Phase III: Summary

In Phase III, between Days 11 and 15 of the Body Reset, you'll have one smoothie, two C-snacks, and two S-meals a day. You'll be alternating Circuits A and B of resistance training while continuing to walk 10,000 steps every day.

The Rest of Your Life

CHAPTER

12

You Then and Now

You did it! You made it through the 15-day reset, and you're probably feeling (and looking) pretty amazing right about now. You're finally ready to start incorporating your healthy new habits into your life for the long haul, embracing a lifestyle change that you can sustain for years to come.

First let's check your progress: Just look at all you've achieved already! In just 15 days, you've lost weight, toned up your body, and saved money without sacrificing any time from your already-packed schedule.

Here's how it works going forward: Like I keep saying, so many diets fail because they fail to take into account how the real world actually works—how busy we are, how stretched our budgets are, how easily discouraged we can become. Once you get to the end of Day 15, you can—and will—keep going. Just continue doing what you've already been doing! The only difference is that now you're able to enjoy two "free" meals a week during which you can eat and drink whatever you want!

That's right, two meals of your choice. Why? Because life isn't about deprivation. It should be enjoyed and it's okay to occasionally eat your favorite foods, as long as you're following this plan for your other meals the rest of the week.

Getting Creative

As you get more confident with your blender (and you'll see that it doesn't take long at all), you can also follow the Build Your Own Smoothie guidelines I lay out starting on page 69, which couldn't be more straightforward: As long as you hit all the major nutritional categories—fiber, protein, healthy fat—you can experiment to your heart's content. Just don't forget that a smoothie without one of these key categories doesn't count as a meal, so if you throw bananas, strawberries, and ice in a blender, you're not getting the protein you need to stay full until the next meal.

When you choose to have your daily smoothie is still entirely up to

Hitting **Reset** Again

Whenever you need to lose a few pounds fast—say, after the holidays or a particularly indulgent long weekend—you can easily reintegrate Phase I or II of the Body Reset, either for 1 day or the full 5 days. Even a temporary reset can serve as a great detox at a moment's notice, without forgoing any essential nutrients. Reverting to Phase I in particular can help you lose weight in a hurry if you have a big event coming up and want to tighten up a bit, or just feel like you need an extra boost.

But the timing is entirely up to you. It really just depends on what type of reset you want and what your body needs at the time. Maybe you will revisit Phase II for a little tweak once a month, or Phase I once a season, just to turn over a new leaf. That's what I like to do: drink three smoothies a day for the first 5 days of summer, fall, and so forth, for a fresh start. However you choose to use it, this plan is always there for you when you need it!

you. I'm always doing 10 things at once from the second I get out of bed, so I generally opt to have my daily smoothie for breakfast, cycling through the red, green, and white smoothies (I *love* the PB&J Smoothie) depending on my mood and what I happen to have in my fridge. The rest of the day I eat as I always have: two meals and two snacks that all contain a healthy blend of fiber, protein, and healthy fat. You can also choose to have your daily smoothie at the time of day that you might be most vulnerable to bingeing.

The one big (and I'm sure welcome) change in this phase is that you'll now get to have two "free" meals a week—that is to say, meals when none of the rules apply.

Bonus Perk: The Free Meal

As your reward for making it through all 15 days (as if your looser-fitting jeans weren't enough), you can now incorporate two weekly "free" meals into your diet. At free meals, you can eat and drink whatever you want. You can enjoy these meals as a Sunday brunch, a Friday night dinner with friends, or date night with your significant other. It's completely up to you.

Why these "free" meals instead of the "cheat day" I included as part of my 5-Factor plan? Well, many popular diets (including mine) have a cheat day, but I've found that just calling it by that name makes people feel compelled to not just indulge but overindulge, and even to abuse their bodies. I've had clients who even wake up extra early on their cheat day so they can have more hours to jam down pancakes and hamburgers and pizza—nope, I am not making this up.

(P.S. Thank you to all my Facebook and Twitter friends—I polled you all and you pretty much unanimously chose two free meals over one cheat day!)

So after much consideration, I've gotten rid of the word "cheat" because you're not really cheating anything; you're just removing the structure of the rest of the week. "Free" can have a multitude of different meanings. Maybe it means that you eat a healthy meal but have dessert, or maybe it means that you have a few drinks with your meal—"free" can mean whatever you want it to mean.

Another advantage of the two free meals over the one cheat day is that dedicating a whole day to cheating meant people felt they had to be completely perfect for the other 6 days, and that's really difficult. Often, people have a social event (or two) during the week, and I don't want them to quit the whole program because it doesn't accommodate their social life. Getting two free meals a week is better for your social life—

and your body. After all, a cheat day means up to three meals and two snacks of cheating, whereas two free meals a week is exactly that: two meals, so it's less than half as much indulging.

This plan is all about lasting years, not days, and I find that too much deprivation and too-stringent regulations can often produce an unwanted backlash. You feel resentful when you are always denying yourself the treats you used to love, so instead of sticking to the straight and narrow, you find yourself bingeing more and more. That's why I'd really prefer that you treat these free meals as special occasions—rewards for how great you are doing—rather than just

Alcohol: **A Few Cautions**

Alcohol has nearly twice the calories of carbohydrates and protein, but that's not my main concern with it. I'm more worried about the enzymatic environment created by consumption of alcohol. When we consume alcohol, our liver has to work overtime to create the enzymes necessary to metabolize it. But our liver is also responsible for metabolizing fat, so when it's working on metabolizing the alcohol, it's not creating the enzymes necessary to burn fat. So, put simply, *when we drink alcohol, our bodies are doing a less efficient job of metabolizing fat.* More obvious, perhaps, and equally pernicious are the behavioral hazards of drinking alcohol: When we're under the influence of booze, we have a tendency to eat with abandon. I consider alcohol a gateway drug of sorts—not necessarily for more drugs but for poor food choices. That said, as I learned when researching *The 5-Factor World Diet*, many of the world's healthiest countries include alcohol as part of their lifestyles, though always in moderation. If you exercise caution and indulge only at your free meals, you can enjoy alcohol without endangering your newly slim waist. So it's fine if alcohol is your splurge, but let it be part of your free meals.

eat an entire box of sugary cereal in front of the television.

Never feel guilty about what you eat at your free meals; after all, you've earned them. Eating badly twice a week is still much healthier than eating sort of badly around the clock. It's the accumulation of carbohydrates and sugars day in and day out that does your body the most harm, not the rare indulgence. So go on out and have fun! And look at it this way: If you're eating 35 times a week (21 meals and 14 snacks) and splurging on just 2 of those, then you are still way ahead of the game.

I've also found that, if you take these free meals in the context of an otherwise healthy diet, you might not find those old junk foods quite as tempting as you once did. You might experience a sugar headache, or indigestion, from the assault of processed foods on your newly pristine body. You'll be less tempted to eat and drink to excess; your body just won't want the same poisons anymore.

So go on and head out to your favorite Mexican restaurant and dig into that chip basket. Have a slice of carrot cake if you so desire; it's your free meal, so there are no limits. You can even have alcohol, though I've offered a few general health reservations about it.

Of course, the bottom line here is that life is meant to be lived, and I'm not going to tell you *anything* you cannot do on your two free meals a week. That's why they're free! You can eat or drink absolutely anything you want, though if you want to keep your alcoholic beverages on the healthier side, I'd suggest avoiding sugary drinks like piña coladas and daiquiris. But regardless, it's YOUR free meal, so go ahead and indulge to your heart's content. Like I said, you've earned it.

> "My sister and I don't think the diets in the past worked for us because we weren't ready and they were just fads. Reading Harley's book and being on his program made us realize that it wasn't a diet at all—it was a lifestyle change. Eating five small meals a day with the protein and fiber we needed was a

great combination with our workouts. Our families were—and still are—amazed by our weight loss. We will tell anyone: It starts in YOUR mind."

—Jamilla and Cherrell Harris, *each lost 9 pounds in 15 days*

Navigating the Rest of Your Life: Tips for Long-Term Success

Plan, plan, and plan some more. I know I'm getting a little repetitive on this subject, but one of the most effective ways to ensure your continued success on this plan is to plot out your mealtimes well ahead of time. Don't leave anything to chance and get into a situation where your blood sugar is so low and your hunger so raging that you will eat everything in sight and then some. If you plan your meals and snacks at intervals of about 3 hours, you are far, far less likely to fall into this trap. But obviously, every day (and every mood) is different, and if you do feel hungry unexpectedly off your usual schedule, reach for a calorie-free beverage to see if that helps alleviate the pangs. And if planning works for you, consider also keeping a food journal, which has been shown to promote weight loss.[1]

Be mindful of why you're eating. Often, we don't eat because we're hungry. We eat because we're stressed or bored or unhappy. The best cure for this vague discontent is activity. If you're spending 4 hours a night watching TV on the couch, you're going to snack more. But if you're spending those same hours gardening in the backyard or playing tennis with an old friend, then by default you're won't be snacking mindlessly quite so often. A nuanced awareness of eating habits, both good and bad, is key to weight-loss success. That's one reason it can help to write down everything you eat or use an app that helps track your daily food intake.

Cover all your bases. Remember, to give your body the fuel it needs to thrive—rather than filling it with a bunch of empty calories that drag you down—you want to hit a few basic categories at every meal or snack: You've got to have fiber, and you've got to have protein. Without those two elements, your body is going to crave more food sooner than it needs it. Whenever you buy packaged foods, check the label to make sure they contain at least 5 grams of fiber and protein and weigh in at under 150 calories per serving.

Slow down—and stop while you're ahead. Get out of the habit of gorging yourself every time you sit down to eat. Chew thoroughly before swallowing, and make an effort to leave a few bites on your plate, just to see if you can. And take a cue from the Japanese, who try to stop eating when they're 80 percent (instead of our habitual 200 percent) full. Instead of lunging for the dessert tray right away, Japanese are raised to wait 5 to 10 minutes to see if they still want food. The vast majority of the time, they don't—and you won't, either. Try it on your next free meal. You might be impressed by your own self-control!

> "My best advice to anyone starting on a journey toward health and wellness is to start right now. Not tomorrow, not Monday, but NOW. Make the commitment and stick to it. This isn't a diet—it's a lifestyle change! While it can be challenging, what better reward is there than a life of health, wellness, and feeling good about your body?"
> —Delia Larson, *lost 11 pounds in 15 days*

Stock up on healthy foods in advance. Knowing what not to buy is one thing, but knowing what TO buy is just as important. I find it helpful to keep my pantry and fridge stocked at all times with healthy staples that I can turn into delicious meals in seconds flat.

- For smoothies: I go through stretches when I stock up on large quantities of spinach, frozen berries, fat-free Greek yogurt, and almonds—all of which I buy in bulk.

- For stir-fries: I always keep a bag of presliced stir-fried veggies in my freezer in case of emergency.

- For scrambles: I buy a big carton of egg whites. For sandwiches, I buy whole grain, high-fiber bread (at least 5 grams of fiber per serving) and I freeze it, making it last longer.

- For salads: I go with fresh veggies, buying whatever's in season or on sale at my local market.

- For soups: I sometimes double or even triple the recipe so that I can freeze extra portions when I'm in a hurry but want to eat something on the plan. This is an especially helpful tip during the winter months. I also buy low-sodium chicken or vegetable bouillon and fibrous vegetables like cauliflower and broccoli to throw in the blender.

Clean house. If you want to stick to this plan, it's a good idea to get rid of all the high-sugar foods in your house. You don't need to be tempted by sweetened cereals and fattening cookies in your life, so why do you have them in your kitchen? Replace anything with the words "hydrogenated" or "high fructose" with delicious whole foods so that you won't fall prey to temptation in weak moments. (We all have them.) Many of the toughest battles take place in the snack-food aisles of the grocery store, so show up with a list and stick to your goals. Having kids is no excuse: They don't need those unhealthy foods, either. Nuts, fruits, and low-fat cheese sticks make a much healthier after-school snack than the usual junk we give our children. If other people in the house insist on keeping junk food around, keep it in a specially designated cupboard, not at eye level.

Order wisely. Yes, you *can* eat whatever you want at your free meals, but try not to leave all your hard-won knowledge about health and nutrition at the restaurant door. In particular, remember that a meal isn't a meal without protein and fiber, so try to keep that in mind when you're scanning the menu of your favorite restaurant. Also, as always, pay attention to portion sizes, which tend to be gigantic everywhere we go these days. Avoid the bread or chip basket if you can—that's one of the big reasons we eat so much (often without even noticing) when we go to restaurants. If you save your appetite for the main event, you might find that you enjoy the food more. Getting in the habit of taking a doggie bag home with you is a great way to save on calories without restricting your favorite foods. Ask for it when you're ordering to limit temptation. Instead of wiping your plate clean, try to save a portion of your meal for lunch the next day, or bring some home for a (sure to be grateful) family member. Don't be afraid to ask for dressing and sauces on the side.

Stick to a schedule. Yep, keeping a consistent schedule is just as important, if not more so, in this lifelong phase. Get into the habit of knowing what you're going to eat beforehand. At the beginning of the week, try to have some idea of when you'll be taking your free meals. Make sure your kitchen is stocked with the foods you need to make a smoothie every day and healthy S-meals and C-snacks the rest of the time. Before going to bed at night, have an idea of what you'll be having when you wake up. The same advance planning that got you through the first 15 days with such ease will be an invaluable resource as you adapt this way of eating to the rest of your life. This chart will guide you through the first 5 days of planning how you'll be eating for many years to come. It should be old hat by this stage!

THE REST OF YOUR LIFE

	Monday	Tuesday	Wednesday	Thursday	Friday
Breakfast	White smoothie	Italian Flag Breakfast Pizza (page 184)	Harley's Potato-Pepper Easy Omelet (page 186)	Herbed Cream Cheese Scramble (page 188)	Red smoothie
Snack 1	Snack	Snack	Snack	Snack	Snack
Lunch	Curried Turkey and Pear Sandwich (page 199)	Red smoothie	Roast Beef and Caramelized Onion Wrap (page 196)	Southwestern Tuna Tortilla Wrap (page 198)	Curried Turkey and Pear Sandwich (page 199)
Snack 2	Snack	Snack	Snack	Snack	Snack
Dinner	S-meal	Free meal	10-Minute Stir-Fry (page 218)	White smoothie	Free meal

Keep it simple! Last but not least, simplicity is the key to success in dieting, so don't make it harder than it has to be. We have complicated everything in our lives way, way too much. Whenever you haven't succeeded on a diet, I would wager that it's because you overcomplicated it (or, more likely, that the diet itself was overcomplicated to begin with). With *The Body Reset Diet,* you'll be having a smoothie a day for the rest of your life—and nothing could be simpler, as you've surely learned by now, than throwing delicious foods into a blender and pressing Start.

Stick to your fitness plan. This is just so, so important, I really can't emphasize it enough. Your fitness plan will be the same as it was during Phase III: As always (do I even need to remind you at this point?), you will keep on walking your 10,000 steps a day, 7 days a week. If you're ready to walk even more to expedite the results, then go for it, but do make sure it's a gradual increase. Going too fast is how you get shin splints, plantar fasciitis, and sore knees. It's not so much a problem of repetitive stress injuries as of diminishing returns. In the long run, moderation always wins out.

Don't forget—while physical activity such as walking burns calories, you also have to do regular resistance training to strengthen and tone your body. To that end, you will continue doing Circuit A 3 days a week and Circuit B 2 days a week. In general, I'd suggest you make an effort to work out Monday through Friday, but really, any 5 days will do as long as you're consistent.

As before, you will slowly graduate from the beginner to the intermediate and advanced circuits as your body gets stronger, and once a month you will add an additional circuit to your workout until you reach three circuits. Many of the more advanced exercisers out there who start out doing three circuits will also increase the level of difficulty of the actual exercise. If you start with the more advanced modifications, then keep adding resistance until you feel your body starting to change. My Web site, www.harleypasternak.com, and my previous books, *The 5-Factor Fitness, The 5-Factor Diet,* and *The 5-Factor World Diet,* are great resources for even more exercises if you feel like you want more variety after several months. Or try my video game, *Harley Pasternak's Hollywood Workout.* Whatever you do, I promise these two simple circuits of four exercises each will transform your body.

The keys to all physical activities are being consistent and doing the least you need to do to see the most results. These circuits I've designed are *the* most efficient way of incorporating regular resistance training. I'm not yelling and screaming at you and demanding you do a million completely impossible Olympic feats. I'm asking you to do a tiny series of easy exercises—but do them 5 DAYS A WEEK, every week, no matter where you are or what else you have going on, so that your body keeps getting better and better.

Keep walking all year round. Not all climates are perfect, and some days walking to work just isn't a feasible option. But you can still get your 10,000 steps in 365 days a year whatever the weather. If it's summer, that might mean getting up before the sun for your daily stroll.

(Or, if you're a night owl, wait till the sun has gone down and get your stroll in later in the evening.) For walks in the middle of the day, bring a bottle of water to keep you cool. In the winter, you're sure to get some good exercise shoveling snow, but that doesn't mean you're off the hook for walking. Stroll up and down the stairs of your office building, or drive to the local mall and power-walk from store to store in between errands. You might have to get a little creative, but I promise it's not that hard to hit 10,000 steps even on the nastiest days of the year!

THE BREAKDOWN

Phase I	Phase II	Phase III	The Rest of Your Life
—Get a pedometer. —Get a pair of proper-fitting shoes. —Walk 10,000 steps/day.	—Continue to walk 10,000 steps/day. —Start a 5-minute resistance circuit (Circuit A), 3 days/week.	—Continue to walk 10,000 steps/day. —Alternate two resistance circuits (Circuits A and B), 5 days/week.	—Continue to walk 10,000 steps/day. —Continue alternating Circuits A and B, 5 days a week. Gradually increase to three circuits at every session. —Enjoy two free meals a week.

Remember: When it comes to exercise, more is not necessarily better. Think of your body as being like a plant: too little sunlight and it withers up; the same goes for too much sunlight. This exercise regimen is our way of striking the optimal balance between too much and too little resistance training. We want to stimulate our body so that it grows stronger, without overstimulating it so that it gets damaged. Our bodies need time to rest and recover to thrive.

Now . . . pat yourself on the back! As long as you incorporate these lessons into your life, I promise that you will remain successful on the plan, and you will love the dramatic changes in your body. So congratulate yourself on coming this far—and I have all the confidence in the world that you'll continue on this path. Because it works, and when you see how your body changes, you will be inspired to keep going.

Trust me, I know exactly where you're coming from: You want to lose weight ASAP without all the typical roadblocks that have arisen over your years of struggling in vain to lose weight. I heard you loud and clear, and I've designed this plan precisely because I understand how urgent your need is to shed pounds immediately—not next week and not next year, but right away. You came to this book because you've tried everything and nothing has worked for you, whether you're a Hollywood starlet or a school teacher and mom of three. I've seen all the many, many reasons diets don't work, and I've addressed, and offered corrections for, every single one of those reasons. I've shown you how to lose weight quickly and easily without sacrificing your health or putting the rest of your life on hold.

This book contains all the answers you need to embrace a healthier—and happier—future, and there's no better moment to start changing your life than right now!

So there you have it: the simplest, safest, and most immediate weight-loss plan ever. And that weight isn't going to come back. This program will teach you how to drop a lot of weight rapidly and—just as important—how to keep it off. You will be amazed at how quickly your body will change, and you definitely won't be the only one who notices!

Appendix A

Glossary of Smoothie Ingredients and Their Benefits

ALMONDS

Expedite weight loss: Researchers found that people eating a diet rich in almonds lost more weight than those on a high-carb diet with the same number of calories. A 24-week study published in the *International Journal of Obesity* found that a low-calorie diet supplemented with almonds boosted weight loss.[1] Low-calorie diets supplemented with almonds, compared to complex carbohydrates, were linked to a 62 percent greater decrease in weight or BMI, a 50 percent greater decrease in waist circumference, and a 56 percent greater decrease in fat mass. Experts believe the heart-healthy monounsaturated fat in almonds helps satisfy the appetite and curb overeating. Researchers at King's College in London found that almonds seem to help stop the absorption of both carbohydrates and the almonds' own fat content into the body, and also that they increased the satisfied feeling of fullness in both men and women.

Improve brainpower: As if almonds need more to recommend them, they also contain phenylalanine, a brain-boosting chemical that aids healthy development of our cognitive functions.

APPLES AND PEARS

Expedite weight loss: A Brazilian study found that women who ate three apples or pears per day lost more weight while dieting than women who did not eat fruit while dieting. And according to another recent study, a substance in apple peels might also protect against obesity.[2]

Boost the immune system: Red apples contain a powerful antioxidant called quercetin. Recent studies have found that quercetin can help boost and fortify the immune system, especially when you're stressed out. Quercetin is also found in grapes.

Protect bones: French researchers found that a flavonoid (a type of antioxidant) called phloridzin present only in apples may protect postmenopausal women from osteoporosis and may also increase bone density.[3] Boron, another ingredient in apples, also strengthens bones.

AVOCADOS

Improve the skin: Avocados are Mother Nature's moisturizer. With their healthy fats and phytonutrients, avocados can help prevent wrinkles by keeping the skin moist, soft, and supple.

Boost eye health: Avocados have more of the carotenoid lutein than any other commonly consumed fruit. Lutein protects against macular degeneration and cataracts, two disabling age-related eye diseases.

Improve nutrient absorption: Avocados contain the antioxidant vitamin E, essential fatty acids, cholesterol-lowering oleic acid, and the heart protectors potassium and folate. But research has also found that, in addition to being filled with nutrients, avocados help us *absorb* nutrients. In one study, when participants ate a salad containing avocados, they absorbed five times the carotenoids (a group of nutrients that includes lycopene and beta-carotene) absorbed by those whose salads didn't include avocados.[4]

BERRIES

Reduce belly bloat: A University of Michigan Cardiovascular Center study suggests that blueberries may help reduce belly fat and risk factors for cardiovascular disease and metabolic syndrome.[5]

Subtract years: According to a Tufts University study,[6] blueberries are one of nature's most powerful antiaging supplements. The antioxidant found in blueberries can prevent oxidative damage, a process that damages your cells and ages you.

Improve eyesight: Blueberries' antioxidant properties can prevent or delay age-related eye problems like cataracts and macular degeneration.

CHIA SEEDS

Expedite weight loss: The essential fatty acids in chia seeds—the survival food of Aztec warriors—help speed up metabolism and promote lean muscle mass. They contain even higher levels of omega-3 fatty acids than salmon and are also high in calcium.

Improve digestion: Chia seeds are also very high in fiber and can add bulk to your diet without adding too many calories. They will help keep food moving through your intestines, which is essential if you want to lose weight.

CINNAMON

Lowers blood sugar: Studies have shown that the almighty cinnamon can help lower blood sugar in people with diabetes and might also prevent insulin resistance, which leads to diabetes and a host of other health problems, in the rest of the population. Adding cinnamon to a high-carb food might actually lessen the impact of the carbohydrate on your blood sugar levels. It's one of the best metabolism-regulating ingredients there is.

Boosts cognitive function: Cinnamon might help counteract complications associated with traumatic brain injury and stroke that cause restricted blood supply to the brain, according to a study by the US Department of Agriculture.[7] And Alzheimer's disease researchers are currently working to understand the role of cinnamon in alleviating the formation of proteins associated with this ravaging disease of the brain.

GREEK YOGURT, FAT-FREE PLAIN

Expedites weight loss: There's growing evidence that high-calcium diets from dairy sources can aid weight loss. A study published in the *International Journal of Obesity* showed that dieters who ate high-calcium yogurt lost 81 percent more belly fat than dieters on a low-calcium diet. And a University of Tennessee study suggested that dieters who ate three servings of yogurt a day lost 22 percent more weight and 61 percent more body fat than those who simply cut calories and didn't add calcium to their eating plan.

Improves hair health: Greek yogurt contains a substantial amount of protein, which is important for hair health. If you are vegetarian or just trying to cut back on meat, eating a portion of Greek yogurt may confer the same protein benefits as eating a serving of meat. *U.S. News & World Report* found that 6 ounces of Greek yogurt has about the same amount of protein as 2 to 3 ounces of lean meat, or about 15 to 20 grams.

(A comparable serving of regular plain yogurt, the same *U.S. News and World Report* story found, contains only 9 grams of protein, which means you'll be hungrier earlier.)[8]

Provides a great alternative to regular yogurt: Greek yogurt doesn't just beat its conventional counterpart when it comes to protein. It's also lower in lactose and lower in sugar, with a much richer texture and *half* the carbs (5 to 8 grams per serving compared with 13 to 17 grams in regular yogurt)—all for roughly the same calorie count.

LIMES

Fight constipation: The high acid levels in limes, as in all citrus fruits, can have a mild laxative effect and help clean out the bowels. But unlike many citrus fruits, limes are very low in calories—and add tremendous flavor.

Fight disease: Limes are much higher in vitamin C than lemons, which means they have a greater concentration of this essential antioxidant that counteracts free radical damage and protects against a wide range of ailments, from heart disease to cancer.

ORANGES

Protect the immune system: Oranges are rich in vitamin C, a key antioxidant that can help protect against immune system deficiencies, cardiovascular disease, prenatal health problems, eye disease, and even skin wrinkling. Vitamin C can even help reverse the free radical damage associated with cancer.

Lower blood pressure: Animal studies have shown that a phytonutrient (or a nutrient found in plants) in oranges, herperidin, can lower both high blood pressure and cholesterol. But this essential ingredient is found only in the peel and white pulp, which means it gets removed during the juicing (but *not* the blending) process.

PROTEIN POWDER

Builds healthy muscles and bones: Protein is an essential part of every meal because without it, your body doesn't have the resources to repair itself. Unlike carbohydrates or fats, protein cannot be stored in the body, and it must be frequently consumed. It supplies your body with the essential amino acids it needs to build nails, hair, and muscles.

Helps improve endurance: Whey protein isolate is absorbed quickly into the body and can improve your stamina and endurance during athletic activities, which is one reason professional athletes are such fans of the protein shake. Whey protein also stimulates the release of serotonin, a hormone that promotes feelings of calmness.

Choosing the
Right Protein Powder

Become a label reader when you're shopping for protein powder. Every serving—which should weigh in at about 15 to 20 grams—should contain less than 2 grams of fat and 2 grams of sugar. As long as at least 90 percent of the calories come from protein, you're in good shape. But what type of protein powder should you get? The options, I admit, can be dizzying. Here are my favorites, but you can experiment and see which powder works best for you. My favorite is Shaklee's instant protein.

- Brown rice
- Dairy (whey or casein)
- Egg white (albumin)
- Pea
- Soy (non-GMO)

Expedites weight loss: The body burns more energy when digesting protein than any other food, and so eating a lot of protein can speed up your metabolism and help you burn off the pounds. Whey protein can also help slow the absorption rate of glucose into the bloodstream.

SPINACH

Provides great caloric efficiency: Remember when I said that our goal is to make every calorie count? Well, spinach and other leafy green vegetables like kale are among the most calorie-efficient foods you can eat. Spinach contains a wide range of anti-inflammatory and antioxidant agents that can fight everything from osteoporosis to cancer—and all for just 7 calories a cup.

Aids digestion: A single cup of spinach contains nearly 20 percent of the Recommended Dietary Allowance of fiber, meaning it can keep the food moving through your system, fighting constipation and keeping your blood sugar level steady.

Delays aging: Spinach is high in vitamin A, which promotes healthy skin by allowing the epidermis to retain moisture. This in turn can combat psoriasis, acne, wrinkles, and other skin conditions. The high iron and folate content of spinach supports the immune system, enhances vision, slows aging, promotes heart health, and improves blood circulation—all of which can help keep you looking and feeling younger longer.

Strengthens bones: The abundance of vitamin K in spinach helps keep your bones strong, especially as you get older. Vitamin K is also essential for maintaining a healthy nervous system. Basically, if your body needs it done, spinach will do it.

Appendix B

C-Snacks

Remember, these snacks should be crunchy and contain a protein. They should all be about 150 calories and contain at least 5 grams of fiber, 5 grams of protein, and *less than* 10 grams of sugar. You can feel free to mix and match, but here are some ideas for both complete snacks and satisfying combos.

Complete Snacks

Air-popped popcorn
Soy nuts (roasted soybeans)
Freeze-dried peas
Shaklee snack bars (1 oz)

Combo Snacks

1½ bags cruncha ma-me
—135 calories, 12 g protein, 5 g fiber

⅔ c raspberries + 8 oz fat-free Greek yogurt
—170 calories, 23 g protein, 6 g fiber

4 Finn Crisp crackers + 2 slices Kraft fat-free cheese
—170 calories, 18 g protein, 5 g fiber

½ c fat-free cottage cheese + ½ c Fiber One cereal + ¼ c blueberries
—160 calories, 15 g protein, 15 g fiber

3 oz fat-free Greek yogurt + ⅓ Tbsp natural peanut butter
    + Gala apple
—160 calories, 10 g protein, 6 g fiber

3 slices turkey breast + 3 Ryvita crackers + 1 tsp mustard
—153 calories, 14 g protein, 5 g fiber

1 large Bosc pear + 1 low-fat cheese stick
—170 calories, 9 g protein, 4 g fiber

¾ c edamame
—143 calories, 13 g protein, 6 g fiber

3 oz lean roast beef + 1½ red bell peppers
—155 calories, 19 g protein, 5 g fiber

1 tall Starbucks latte with fat-free milk + 1 apple
—154 calories, <1 g protein, 2.4 g fiber

5 ribs celery + 1 Tbsp peanut butter
—155 calories, 7 g protein, 6 g fiber

2 whole grain Ryvita crackers + 3 Tbsp hummus
140 calories, 5 g protein, 6 g fiber

1 apple + 3 turkey slices
—155 calories, 11 g protein, 5 g fiber

1 pear + 2 oz sliced lean roast beef
—165 calories, 14 g protein, 5 g fiber

1 cucumber + 3 oz smoked salmon + 1 tomato
—165 calories, 19 g protein, 4 g fiber

3 Finn Crisp crackers + 1 Tbsp almond butter
—155 calories, 5 g protein, 5 g fiber

2 Kraft fat-free cheese slices + 3 Kavli Golden Rye crispbreads
—140 calories, 11 g protein, 6 g fiber

2 Laughing Cow Light cheese triangles + 5 Grissol multigrain
   Melba Toast crackers
—170 calories, 7 g protein, 5 g fiber

Appendix C

S-Meal Recipes

SCRAMBLES

If you like, you can substitute a whole egg for one of the egg whites after the first 15 days. Just remember, that will add more fat and calories to the meal.

Italian Flag Breakfast Pizza

Serves 1

For the fluffiest scramble, give the egg whites a good strong whisk before adding them to the pan.

COOKING TIP: It's okay to pile the spinach high—it will wilt.

3   egg whites or 6 tablespoons liquid egg substitute

     Salt and black pepper

3   cherry tomatoes, halved

1   whole wheat pita

1   cup baby spinach

1   ounce shredded or sliced part-skim mozzarella cheese

1. Preheat the broiler. Line a baking pan with foil. Place the pan under the broiler to warm it.

2. Coat a small nonstick skillet with cooking spray and place it over medium-high heat. In a small bowl, whisk together the egg whites, salt, and pepper. Cook the egg mixture in the hot skillet for 30 seconds, stirring constantly. Remove from the heat and stir in the tomatoes.

3. Remove the baking pan from the oven. Place the pita on the pan and top it with the spinach, the egg mixture, and the cheese. Season to taste with additional salt and pepper. Broil for 2 minutes, or until the eggs are set and the pita is golden.

Nutrition Info
Calories: 320
Total Fat: 7 grams
Carbs: 37 grams
Protein: 26 grams
Fiber: 7 grams

Harley's Potato-Pepper Easy Omelet

Serves 1

Omelets the easy way! Use a rubber spatula to push and form the omelet in the pan as it cooks—no tricky folding required.

TECHNIQUE TIP: Leave the skin on the potato for added flavor. Just be sure to use a white, or boiling, potato—not a baking, or Idaho, potato.

1	potato, unpeeled, halved and thinly sliced
½	red bell pepper, thinly sliced
½	small onion, thinly sliced
	Salt and black pepper
5	egg whites or 10 tablespoons liquid egg substitute
1	tablespoon shredded Cheddar cheese
1	slice double-fiber whole wheat bread

1. Coat a small nonstick skillet with cooking spray and place it over medium heat. Add the potato, bell pepper, and onion and season them with the salt and pepper. Cook for 8 to 10 minutes, stirring frequently, or until the vegetables soften and are lightly browned.

2. Pour the egg whites into the skillet, gently coating the vegetable mixture with them. Using a spatula, press down on the omelet to flatten it as it cooks. Cook for 1 minute, or until just set. Use the spatula to fold the omelet in half and push it to one-half of the pan, forming a crescent shape. Sprinkle the top with cheese. Cover the skillet for 30 seconds to melt the cheese. Meanwhile, toast the bread.

3. Slide the omelet onto a serving plate. Season to taste with additional salt and pepper. Serve the omelet with the toast.

Nutrition Info
Calories: 355
Total Fat: 5 grams
Carbs: 57 grams
Protein: 29 grams
Fiber: 12 grams

Herbed Cream Cheese Scramble

Serves 1

This creamy scramble cooks in seconds, making this a perfect workday morning meal.

TECHNIQUE TIP: Smoked salmon has such an intense flavor that you only need a small amount!

1   ounce reduced-fat cream cheese, at room temperature

1   tablespoon chopped fresh dill

1   tablespoon chopped fresh chives

   Salt

4   egg whites or 8 tablespoons liquid egg substitute

   Black pepper

2   slices double-fiber whole wheat bread

2   ounces smoked salmon, thinly sliced

1. In a small bowl, mash the cream cheese, dill, and chives until combined. Stir in a pinch of salt. Set aside.
2. Coat a small skillet with cooking spray and place it over medium heat. In a small bowl, whisk the egg whites, additional salt, and pepper. Cook the egg mixture in the hot pan, stirring frequently, until almost set. Meanwhile, toast the bread.
3. Remove the scrambled eggs from the heat. Fold in the reserved cream cheese mixture and the salmon. Serve with the toast.

Nutrition Info
Calories: 300
Total Fat: 9 grams
Carbs: 32 grams
Protein: 33 grams
Fiber: 14 grams

Sweet Potato Hash with Chives

Serves 1

Hearty, healthy, homey—a perfect winter weather breakfast.

COOKING TIP: For quick cooking, it's important to cut the potato and bell pepper into small cubes.

1   sweet potato, peeled and finely chopped

1   small onion, chopped

1   red bell pepper, finely chopped

    Salt and black pepper

4   egg whites or 8 tablespoons liquid egg substitute

½   teaspoon ground paprika

    Fresh chives, for garnish

1. In a shallow microwave-safe bowl, place the sweet potatoes and just enough water to cover. Cover the bowl and microwave on high for 4 minutes, or until the sweet potatoes are tender. Drain.

2. Coat a large nonstick skillet with cooking spray and place it over medium heat. Add the onion, bell pepper, and sweet potatoes. Season with the salt and pepper and cook for 5 minutes, stirring frequently, or until tender. Increase the heat to medium-high and cook for 5 more minutes, or until crisp. Scrape the hash onto a serving plate and cover it to keep it warm.

3. In a bowl, whisk the egg whites. Add the egg whites to the hot skillet and reduce the heat to medium. Quickly scramble the eggs to desired doneness. Spoon the eggs atop the hash. Season to taste with additional salt and pepper and the paprika. Garnish with the chives.

Nutrition Info
Calories: 340
Total Fat: 3 grams
Carbs: 60 grams
Protein: 23 grams
Fiber: 12 grams

Harley's Hearty Egg Muffin

Serves 1

A fast-food dish takes on a healthier profile by using whole wheat muffins and egg whites and adding savory mushrooms.

COOKING TIP: Fresh thyme is a nice addition to the mushrooms—but if you don't have any, the dish is still delicious without it.

2	tablespoons chopped shallot or onion
5	white mushrooms, sliced
	Salt and black pepper
	Chopped fresh thyme
4	egg whites or 8 tablespoons liquid egg substitute
1	whole wheat English muffin
2	tablespoons (1/2 ounce) shredded Cheddar cheese

1. Coat a small nonstick skillet with cooking spray and place it over medium-low heat. Cook the shallot or onion and mushrooms for 4 minutes, stirring frequently, or until the mushrooms give off their juices and are softened and cooked through. Season to taste with the salt, pepper, and thyme. Scrape the mixture into a bowl.

2. Coat the same skillet with additional cooking spray and place it over medium heat. In a bowl, whisk the egg whites. Scramble the egg whites in the hot pan until they are set. Meanwhile, toast the English muffin.

3. On a serving plate, top each muffin half with half of the eggs and half of the mushroom mixture. Sprinkle with the cheese and cover briefly with foil to melt the cheese.

Nutrition Info
Calories: 290
Total Fat: 7 grams
Carbs: 35 grams
Protein: 28 grams
Fiber: 7 grams

Breakfast Burrito I   Serves 2

Burritos are my favorite "on the go" breakfast. They are very filling and easy to make.

- 2 egg whites or ¼ cup liquid egg substitute
- 1 teaspoon onion powder
- 2 teaspoons taco seasoning mix
-    Salt and cracked black pepper
- 1 cup fat-free ricotta cheese
- 4 whole grain or whole wheat tortillas
- 4 cups diced tomatoes
- 8 cups spinach leaves

1. Coat a medium nonstick skillet with cooking spray and place it over medium heat. Cook the mushrooms until they turn golden. Add the egg whites, onion powder, taco seasoning mix, and salt and pepper to taste. Stir in the cheese and cook, stirring frequently, until the eggs are fully cooked. Set aside.

2. Microwave each tortilla on high for 20 seconds, then place it on a cutting board. Place the scrambled eggs, tomatoes, and spinach in the center of each tortilla. Roll tightly into a burrito shape and keep warm.

3. On a cutting board, slice each burrito in half. Serve while hot.

Nutrition Info
Calories: 374
Total Fat: 4 grams
Carbs: 56 grams
Protein: 34 grams
Fiber: 11 grams

Breakfast Burrito II   Serves 2

Living in LA, I've learned to love Mexican food. This is my healthy spin on an egg burrito.

16   egg whites or 2 cups liquid egg substitute

Salt and black pepper

2   large whole grain or whole wheat tortillas

1¼ cups refried beans

¼   cup (1 ounce) shredded fat-free Cheddar cheese

2   cups mild or spicy salsa

1. Coat a medium nonstick skillet with cooking spray and place it over medium heat. Pour in the egg whites and salt and pepper to taste and cook, stirring frequently, 1½ minutes or until cooked through. Set aside.

2. Microwave the tortillas on high for 15 seconds. Spread the refried beans on the tortillas and spoon the scrambled eggs over the beans. Sprinkle the cheese on top of the eggs and roll the tortillas tightly into a burrito shape.

3. Cut each burrito in half. Spoon the salsa over the burritos or serve the salsa on the side.

Nutrition Info
Calories: 465
Total Fat: 3 grams
Carbs: 62 grams
Protein: 46 grams
Fiber: 15 grams

Sweet Potato Home Fries and Eggs

Serves 2

Like your typical diner breakfast—only healthier!

Cooking tip: If fat-free Cheddar cheese is difficult to find, you may replace it with shredded part-skim mozzarella.

1¼ pounds sweet potatoes

½ cup finely chopped Spanish onions

2 bell peppers, finely chopped

1 teaspoon ground paprika

1½ teaspoons garlic powder

1 teaspoon red-pepper flakes

8 egg whites or 1 cup liquid egg substitute

1 cup (4 ounces) shredded fat-free Cheddar cheese

   Salt and cracked black pepper

1. Microwave the sweet potatoes on high for 3 minutes. Let cool somewhat, then peel and finely chop them.

2. Coat a large nonstick pan with cooking spray and place it over medium heat. Cook the onions for 1 minute, stirring frequently, and then add the bell peppers and sweet potato. Season with the paprika, garlic powder, and red-pepper flakes, toss gently, and set side.

3. Coat a small nonstick pan with cooking spray and place it over medium heat. Cook the egg whites, stirring frequently. Add the cheese. Spoon onto plate with home fries and season with salt and pepper to taste.

Nutrition Info
Calories: 390
Total Fat: 1 gram
Carbs: 60 grams
Protein: 36 grams
Fiber: 8 grams

Open-Faced Egg and Bacon Sandwich Serves 2

Perhaps the most popular breakfast recipe I've developed to date.

Cooking tip: If you can't find fat-free Cheddar cheese, you may substitute shredded, part-skim mozzarella.

- 2 strips turkey bacon
- 10 egg whites or 1¼ cups liquid egg substitute
  Salt and black pepper
- 4 slices whole grain bread
- ½ cup (2 ounces) shredded fat-free Cheddar cheese
- 1¼ cups plum tomatoes, seeded and finely chopped

1. Microwave the turkey bacon strips on high for 3 to 4 minutes or until crispy. Set them aside to cool.
2. Coat a medium nonstick pan with cooking spray and place it over medium heat. Add the egg whites and season them to taste with the salt and pepper. Cook, stirring frequently, 1½ minutes or until the eggs are not runny. Set aside. Meanwhile, toast the bread.
3. Spoon the scrambled eggs on top of each piece of toast. Top with the cheese, turkey bacon, and tomatoes.

Nutrition Info
Calories: 412
Total Fat: 6 grams
Carbs: 56 grams
Protein: 36 grams
Fiber: 8 grams

SANDWICHES

The components of the sandwiches are completely interchangeable—the caramelized onions of the Roast Beef and Caramelized Onion Wrap would be great with the sliced chicken in the Tzatziki Chicken Flatbread or sliced turkey in the Curried Turkey and Pear Sandwich. And the tzatziki sauce in the Tzatziki Chicken Flatbread would also be delicious with the turkey or roast beef, and so on. As long as you have the basic sauces and fillings down, you can mix and match as you like.

Roast Beef and Caramelized Onion Wrap

Serves 1

Roast beef, creamy horseradish, onion, and watercress are a classic sandwich flavor combination.

TECHNIQUE TIP: Because so little oil is used here, it's important to keep stirring the onions as they cook—you want them to be soft and golden.

1   small onion, thinly sliced

1   whole wheat flatbread

1   teaspoon prepared horseradish

1   tablespoon reduced-fat mayonnaise

3   ounces sliced roast beef

1   cup coarsely chopped watercress

1. Coat a small nonstick skillet with cooking spray and place it over medium-low heat. Add the onion. Reduce the heat to low and cook for 8 minutes, stirring frequently, until the onion is golden.

2. Meanwhile, in a toaster oven or an oven preheated to 350ºF, warm the flatbread. In a small cup, combine the horseradish and mayonnaise. Spread the horseradish mixture on the warm flatbread. Top it with the roast beef, onion, and watercress and roll it up to make a wrap.

Nutrition Info
Calories: 305
Total Fat: 7 grams
Carbs: 38 grams
Protein: 27 grams
Fiber: 9 grams

Lemon Ricotta Edamame Crostini

Serves 1

This pretty plate makes a perfect lunch on a warm day. It also works as an elegant appetizer for your next cocktail party.

FLAVOR TIP: Don't skip the lemon peel—it adds a blast of lemon flavor.

- $\frac{1}{3}$ cup frozen edamame, thawed
- 2 ounces part-skim ricotta cheese
- $\frac{1}{2}$ teaspoon grated lemon peel
- $\frac{1}{2}$ teaspoon fresh lemon juice
- Chopped parsley
- Salt and black pepper
- 2 slices double-fiber whole wheat bread
- $\frac{1}{2}$ cup baby arugula

1. In a small saucepan, cook the edamame according to package directions. In a small bowl, combine the cheese, lemon peel, lemon juice, and parsley. Season to taste with the salt and pepper.

2. Meanwhile, toast the bread. Slather the bread with the ricotta mixture, then mound it with the edamame and arugula.

Nutrition Info
Calories: 285
Total Fat: 9 grams
Carbs: 37 grams
Protein: 23 grams
Fiber: 15 grams

Southwestern Tuna Tortilla Wrap

Serves 2

Salsa is not just for dipping. Tailor the spiciness of your sandwich filling by selecting mild or hot varieties of salsa.

SERVING TIP: Unlike our other sandwich recipes, this one serves 2, so save the second one for lunch tomorrow!

6	tablespoons mild or medium salsa
2	tablespoons reduced-fat mayonnaise
1	tablespoon fresh lime juice
2	tablespoons chopped fresh cilantro
1	can (6 ounces) albacore tuna, packed in water
	Salt and black pepper
	Ground cumin
2	whole wheat tortillas
1	cup shredded romaine lettuce

In a medium bowl, stir the salsa, mayonnaise, lime juice, and cilantro until combined. Fold in the tuna and season to taste with the salt, pepper, and cumin. Mound the tuna mixture onto the tortillas. Top with the lettuce. Carefully roll up the tortillas to make 2 wraps.

Nutrition Info
Calories: 240
Total Fat: 6 grams
Carbs: 25 grams
Protein: 29 grams
Fiber: 14 grams

Curried Turkey and Pear Sandwich

Serves 1

Pears are a fiber-rich snack and a sweet addition to this sandwich.

SUBSTITUTION TIP: Pears out of season? Use an apple instead.

- ½ ounce fat-free plain Greek yogurt

  Salt and black pepper
- ¼ teaspoon curry powder
- 2 slices double-fiber whole grain bread
- 3 ounces sliced turkey
- 1 pear, unpeeled and thinly sliced
- 1 leaf red leaf or romaine lettuce

In a small bowl, whisk together the yogurt, salt and pepper to taste, and curry powder until combined. Spread the curried yogurt on 1 slice of bread. Layer the turkey, pear, and lettuce atop the curried yogurt and top with the second slice of bread.

Nutrition Info
Calories: 280
Total Fat: 3 grams
Carbs: 50 grams
Protein: 20 grams
Fiber: 14 grams

Tzatziki Chicken Flatbread

Serves 1

Tzatziki is a Greek or Turkish cucumber yogurt sauce. Here it's deconstructed in an easy chicken salad sandwich.

SHOPPING TIP: Be sure to check the Nutrition Facts when selecting a flatbread at the supermarket. Look for a brand with a high fiber content.

1	teaspoon extra-virgin olive oil
2	teaspoons fresh lemon juice
	Salt and black pepper
½	small cucumber, halved and very thinly sliced
1	small tomato, chopped
3	ounces cooked boneless, skinless chicken breast, sliced
1	tablespoon chopped fresh dill
1	whole wheat flatbread
1	ounce fat-free plain Greek yogurt

In a small bowl, whisk together the oil, lemon juice, and salt and pepper to taste. Add the cucumber, tomato, chicken, and dill and toss to coat. Meanwhile, in a toaster oven or conventional oven preheated to 350°F, warm the flatbread. Pile the chicken salad atop the flatbread. Top with the yogurt.

Nutrition Info
Calories: 325
Total Fat: 10 grams
Carbs: 25 grams
Protein: 39 grams
Fiber: 10 grams

Open-Faced Chicken and Caramelized Onion Sandwich

Serves 2

Thin-sliced boneless, skinless chicken breasts, sometimes called cutlets, cook in just minutes. Substitute a precooked chicken breast if you like.

COOKING TIP: Cooking sliced onions at a low heat for a long time caramelizes their natural sugars and lends a sweetness to the sandwich topping.

1   large onion, halved and very thinly sliced (about 3 cups)

1   tablespoon balsamic vinegar

    Salt and pepper

2   (2½-ounce) boneless, skinless chicken breast halves (cutlets), thinly sliced

2   (8") whole grain baguette halves

1. Coat a large nonstick skillet with cooking spray and place it over medium-low heat. Cook the onions for 15 minutes, stirring frequently. Add up to 2 tablespoons water and reduce the heat if the onions begin to scorch. Add the vinegar and the salt to taste. Cook, stirring frequently, 4 minutes longer or until golden. Scrape the onions onto a plate.

2. Coat the same skillet with additional cooking spray and place it over medium heat. Season the chicken with salt and pepper to taste and cook for 4 minutes per side, until cooked through.

3. Meanwhile, toast the baguette halves. Top each with a warm chicken breast and half the onions.

Nutrition Info
Calories: 480
Total Fat: 13 grams
Carbs: 70 grams
Protein: 20 grams
Fiber: 8 grams

Greek Tuna Melt

The temperate climate of Greece means tomatoes can be eaten throughout much of the year. They make a perfect partner for tuna and salty feta cheese, with pita wedges for scooping.

1	can (6 ounces) white albacore tuna packed in water, drained
1	teaspoon olive oil
1	teaspoon red wine vinegar
	Salt and black pepper
1	large tomato, thinly sliced
¼	cup (1 ounce) reduced-fat feta cheese, crumbled
1	teaspoon chopped fresh oregano
2	whole grain pitas, cut into wedges

1. In a small bowl, toss the tuna with the oil, vinegar, and salt and pepper to taste.

2. On a large microwave-safe plate, arrange the tomato slices so that they are slightly overlapping. Sprinkle the tomatoes with the tuna mixture and the feta cheese. Microwave on high for 2 minutes, or until the cheese bubbles and the tuna is warmed through. Sprinkle with the oregano. Serve hot with the pita wedges.

Nutrition Info
Calories: 230
Total Fat: 6 grams
Carbs: 18 grams
Protein: 26 grams
Fiber: 3 grams

Homemade Gyros

Serves 2

Growing up in Toronto, I used to visit our local Greek area for my favorite Gyros lunch.

1	teaspoon ground paprika
1/2	teaspoon fresh oregano or 1/4 teaspoon dried
	Salt and black pepper
3/4	pound boneless pork loin, thinly sliced
1/2	teaspoon white wine vinegar
2	whole grain pitas
1/4	cup prepared tzatziki (see Tzatziki Chicken Flatbread, page 200)
1/2	cup thinly sliced red onion
1	tomato, thinly sliced

1. Preheat the oven to 300°F. In a small bowl, combine the paprika, oregano, salt, and pepper.

2. Use a mallet or the bottom of a saucepan to pound the pork slices to less than 1/4" thick. Lay the pork slices in a glass 13" x 9" baking pan. Sprinkle with the paprika mixture, then drizzle with the vinegar until the pork is moist. Refrigerate for 30 minutes.

3. Coat a large nonstick skillet with cooking spray and place it over high heat. Cook the pork for 3 minutes per side, until browned and cooked through.

4. Wrap the pitas in foil and warm them in the oven for 15 minutes. Make 2 gyros by stacking the pork, tzatziki, onion, and tomato on the warm pitas.

Nutrition Info

Calories: 370
Total Fat: 15 grams
Carbs: 21 grams
Protein: 39 grams
Fiber: 3 grams

SOUPS

Creamy Black Bean and Pumpkin Soup

Serves 2

The flavors of this soup are so rich you'd never guess that the beans and pumpkin come from a can!

SERVING TIP: This soup will keep for several days in the refrigerator. You may need to add some liquid when you reheat it.

- 2   cups rinsed and drained canned black beans
- ½   can (15 ounces) pumpkin (not pumpkin pie mix)
- ½   cup chopped tomatoes (canned or fresh)
- ½   cup chopped onion
-       Salt and black pepper
-       Ground cumin
- 1   can (14.5 ounces) reduced-sodium chicken broth
- 1   tablespoon sherry or red wine vinegar
- 1   tablespoon pumpkin seeds, for garnish

1. In a blender, puree the beans, pumpkin, and tomatoes.

2. Coat a medium saucepan with cooking spray and place it over medium heat. Cook the onion for 4 minutes, stirring frequently, until softened. Season to taste with the salt, pepper, and cumin.

3. Add the bean puree and broth to the pan. Bring to a simmer and cook for 20 minutes, stirring occasionally. The soup will be thick. Remove from the heat and stir in the sherry or vinegar. Garnish the soup with the pumpkin seeds.

Nutrition Info
Calories: 390
Total Fat: 3 grams
Carbs: 67 grams
Protein: 25 grams
Fiber: 16 grams

Sunset Squash Soup

Serves 2

Since this recipe makes 2 servings, save half of it to bring to work for lunch.

SHOPPING TIP: Look for precut squash in the produce section.

1   small onion, chopped

     Salt and black pepper

2   cups cubed butternut squash (about ½ squash)

½   can (8 ounces) diced tomatoes

     Pinch of chopped fresh or dried thyme

2½   cups reduced-sodium chicken broth

1½   cups rinsed and drained canned white beans

2   cups baby spinach

2   tablespoons grated Parmesan, for garnish

1. Coat a medium saucepan with cooking spray and place it over medium–low heat. Add the onion and season it to taste with the salt and pepper. Cook for 4 minutes, stirring frequently, until softened.

2. Add the squash, tomatoes, and thyme. Cook for 2 minutes, stirring, to combine the flavors. Add the broth. Increase the heat to high and bring to a simmer. Cook for 15 to 20 minutes, stirring occasionally, until the squash is tender. Add the beans and spinach and cook 3 minutes more, or until warmed through. Garnish servings of the soup with the Parmesan.

Nutrition Info

Calories: 340
Total Fat: 3 grams
Carbs: 68 grams
Protein: 44 grams
Fiber: 17 grams

Winter's Day Beef with Barley Soup

Barley is traditionally used in beef soups, but feel free to substitute your favorite whole grain.

COOKING TIP: Browning the beef adds flavor to the soup, so don't skip this step.

- ½   cup pearl barley
- 1½   cups water
-       Salt
- ½   medium onion, chopped
- 1   cup sliced carrots
-       Black pepper
- 1½   cups sliced mushrooms (about 8)
- ½   cup chopped fresh or canned tomatoes
- 4   ounces top round steak, sliced
-       Chopped fresh thyme
- 3   cups reduced-sodium chicken broth
- 2   slices double-fiber whole wheat bread

1. In a medium saucepan, combine the barley with the water and a pinch of salt. Bring to a boil over high heat. Reduce the heat to low, cover, and cook for 40 minutes, or until the barley is tender and most of the liquid is absorbed. Fluff with a fork.

2. Coat another medium saucepan with cooking spray and place it over medium heat. Add the onion and carrots, season to taste with salt and pepper, and cook for 3 minutes, or until softened. Reduce the heat to low. Add the mushrooms and tomatoes and cook for 6 minutes, stirring frequently, or until the mushrooms have released their liquid. Stir in the steak and thyme and cook for 30 seconds more.

3. Add the broth and bring the soup to a simmer. Cook for 10 minutes to combine the flavors. Stir in the barley and cook until warmed through and thickened. Meanwhile, toast the bread. Serve the soup with the toast.

Nutrition Info
Calories: 350
Total Fat: 5 grams
Carbs: 56 grams
Protein: 27 grams
Fiber: 11 grams

Homestyle Chicken Soup

Serves 2

*Homemade soup is easy if you are able to pick up
a rotisserie chicken at your supermarket. Just make sure
to use the meat only, not the skin.*

SERVING TIP: Serve with some toasted bread to sop up the
rich broth.

1	cup chopped carrots
½	cup chopped onion
4	cups reduced-sodium chicken broth
1¼	cups cooked brown rice
1	cup chopped cooked boneless, skinless chicken breast
½	cup frozen green peas, thawed
1	slice double-fiber whole wheat bread
2	tablespoons chopped fresh dill, for garnish

1. Coat a medium saucepan with cooking spray and place it over medium heat. Cook the carrots and onion for 5 minutes, stirring frequently, until softened. Add the broth. Increase the heat and bring to a simmer. Cook for 15 minutes to blend the flavors and cook the carrots.

2. Stir in the rice, chicken, and peas. Heat until warmed through. Meanwhile, toast the bread. Garnish servings of the soup with the dill. Cut the toast in half and serve it with the soup.

Nutrition Info
Calories: 335
Total Fat: 4 grams
Carbs: 46 grams
Protein: 26 grams
Fiber: 8 grams

Golden Split Pea Soup

Serves 2

Pea soup is incredibly high in protein and fiber.
It tastes hearty but is still light on your waistline.

½   teaspoon olive oil

2   carrots, chopped

1   small onion, chopped

1   rib celery, chopped

Salt and black pepper

1   cup green or yellow split peas

½   well-rinsed ham hock

1   teaspoon fresh thyme

3   cups reduced-sodium chicken or vegetable broth

2   slices rye or whole grain bread

1. In a medium saucepan over medium–low heat, warm the oil. Add the carrots, onion, and celery. Season with salt and pepper to taste and cook for 4 minutes, stirring frequently. Add the split peas, ham hock, thyme, and broth. Bring to a simmer, then reduce the heat and cook for 40 minutes, stirring frequently, adding up to 1 cup of water to maintain a soupy consistency.

2. Using a mug, remove about half of the soup. Puree it in a blender. (Alternatively, puree all of the soup in the pot with an immersion blender.) Remove the ham hock and chop ¼ cup of meat from the bone. (Discard the bone.) Return the pureed soup and chopped ham to the pot and warm through. Meanwhile, toast the bread and cut it into triangles. Season the soup to taste with additional salt and pepper and serve it with the toast.

Nutrition Info
Calories: 370
Total Fat: 11g grams
Carbs: 25 grams
Protein: 44 grams
Fiber: 12 grams

SALADS

Black Bean and Lime Mango Salad

Serves 1

For added flavor and color, serve this colorful salad on a bed of chopped lettuce or baby arugula.

INGREDIENT TIP: Use fresh mango if it's in season; otherwise, substitute thawed frozen chopped mango.

1	teaspoon grated lime peel
3	tablespoons fresh lime juice
1	teaspoon extra-virgin olive oil
1	cup rinsed and drained canned black beans
1/2	cup chopped cucumber
1/2	cup chopped fresh mango
1/4	cup chopped avocado
	Salt and black pepper
	Ground cumin

In a medium serving bowl, whisk the lime peel, lime juice, and oil until blended. Add the beans, cucumber, mango, and avocado and toss to coat. Season to taste with salt, pepper, and cumin.

Nutrition Info
Calories: 390
Total Fat: 10 grams
Carbs: 59 grams
Protein: 19 grams
Fiber: 22 grams

Grilled Steak and Baby Spinach Salad

Serves 1

This is a healthier version of a fancy bistro salad—bursting with texture and flavor. Make it tonight!

SHOPPING TIP: We recommend intensely flavored extra-virgin olive oil for salads. Reach for less expensive regular olive oil for cooked dishes.

- 2 ounces top round steak

  Salt and black pepper
- 2 teaspoons balsamic vinegar
- 1 teaspoon extra-virgin olive oil
- 2 cups baby spinach leaves
- 1/2 head fennel, cored and very thinly sliced
- 1/2 cup halved red grapes
- 10 almonds, chopped, for garnish
- 1 whole wheat flatbread

1. Preheat a grill or grill pan over high heat. Season the steak to taste with the salt and pepper. Grill the steak for 5 minutes on each side, or until a thermometer inserted in the center registers 145°F for medium-rare/160°F for medium/165°F for well-done. Let stand for 10 minutes before slicing.

2. Meanwhile, in a serving bowl, whisk the vinegar and oil until blended.

3. Add the spinach, fennel, and grapes to the bowl, tossing to coat. Thinly slice the steak. Add it to the bowl and toss again. Garnish with the almonds. Serve with the flatbread.

Nutrition Info
Calories: 355
Total Fat: 11 grams
Carbs: 37 grams
Protein: 32 grams
Fiber: 13 grams

Dijon Lentil Salad with Baby Spinach

Serves 1

This is one of those magical dishes that can be served warm, at room temperature, or chilled, making it a great bring-to-work lunch option.

COOKING TIP: Cooking time will vary depending on the type of lentils used. If you can find the tiny lentils de Puy, they will cook in 20 minutes. Conventional lentils will take closer to 25 minutes.

2   tablespoons finely chopped shallot or onion

½   cup dried lentils (preferably small French de Puy)

2½ cups water

1   teaspoon extra-virgin olive oil

2   teaspoons Dijon mustard

2   teaspoons red wine vinegar

     Salt and black pepper

1   cup baby spinach

1. Coat a medium nonstick saucepan with cooking spray and place it over medium heat. Cook the shallot or onion for 2 minutes, stirring, until lightly browned. Add the lentils and water and bring to a simmer. Lower the heat and cook for 20 to 25 minutes, adding water if needed, until just tender. Drain, if needed.

2. Meanwhile, in a serving bowl, whisk together the oil, mustard, and vinegar. Stir in the warm lentil mixture. Season with the salt and pepper. Line a shallow bowl with the spinach. Mound the lentils on top and serve.

Nutrition Info
Calories: 300
Total Fat: 5 grams
Carbs: 42 grams
Protein: 20 grams
Fiber: 17 grams

Chicken and Summer Squash Salad with Buttermilk Dressing Serves 2

Who needs a heavy mayonnaise-based potato salad when you can have something like this?

TECHNIQUE TIP: For best flavor, slice the zucchini as thinly as possible.

- 3   tablespoons reduced-fat buttermilk
- 1   tablespoon white wine vinegar
- 1   tablespoon chopped fresh dill
     Salt and black pepper
- 1   small zucchini, halved and sliced paper-thin
- 1   cup halved cherry tomatoes
- ¾   cup chopped cooked boneless, skinless chicken breast
- 2   cups baby arugula

In a medium serving bowl, whisk the buttermilk, vinegar, dill, salt, and pepper until blended. Fold in the zucchini, tomatoes, and chicken. Serve on a bed of the arugula.

Nutrition Info
Calories: 320
Total Fat: 5 grams
Carbs: 31 grams
Protein: 42 grams
Fiber: 9 grams

Lemon Quinoa with Spring Vegetables

Serves 1

Use any combination of spring vegetable: asparagus, green peas, snap peas, scallions. The steaming time should be about the same.

PREP TIP: Some sugar snap peas have a tough string running along the top of the pod. To remove it, snap off the leaf end and pull the string.

2	tablespoons fresh lemon juice
1	clove garlic, minced
1½	cups water
⅓	cup quinoa
1	cup chopped spring vegetables, fresh or frozen (asparagus spears, snap peas, scallions, whole green peas)
½	cup rinsed and drained canned chickpeas
	Salt and black pepper
¼	cup chopped parsley, for garnish

1. In a medium serving bowl, whisk the lemon juice and garlic.
2. In a small saucepan, bring the water to a boil. Add the quinoa, cover, and cook for 7 minutes. Uncover the pan, place the vegetables in a colander or steamer basket, and set it over the cooking quinoa. Cook an additional 5 minutes, or until the vegetables are crisp-tender and the quinoa is tender. Transfer the vegetables to the bowl with the lemon juice and garlic.
3. Fold the warm quinoa and the chickpeas into the bowl. Season to taste with salt and pepper. Garnish with the parsley.

Nutrition Info
Calories: 390
Total Fat: 6 grams
Carbs: 67 grams
Protein: 20 grams
Fiber: 15 grams

Easy Niçoise Salad

Serves 2

This dish is not only delicious, it's truly beautiful when plated thoughtfully.

4	ounces green beans, trimmed and halved
1	can (6 ounces) white albacore tuna packed in water, drained
¼	cup light red wine vinegar
	Salt
4	cups baby lettuce leaves
1	medium tomato, cored and thinly sliced
2	hard-cooked eggs, yolks discarded
4	thin slices whole wheat baguette

1. Bring a small saucepan of water to a boil over high heat. Cook the beans for 3 minutes or until the beans are tender–crisp. Drain and rinse with cool water.
2. In a small bowl, mix the tuna and 2 tablespoons of the vinegar until combined. Season to taste with salt.
3. On a medium platter, arrange the lettuce, tomato slices, beans, and tuna. Drizzle the entire salad with the remaining vinegar. Slice the egg whites and arrange them on the platter. Serve with the baguette.

Nutrition Info
Calories: 360
Total Fat: 8 grams
Carbs: 38 grams
Protein: 33 grams
Fiber: 7 grams

Mexican Chicken Salad with Spicy Salsa Dressing

Serves 2

No cooking necessary! I love this salad because of the easy prep and the way it tastes.

1	teaspoon fajita seasoning mix
	Pinch of ground cumin
	Salt and black pepper
6	ounces boneless, skinless chicken breast
1	cup fat-free sour cream
1	cup mild or hot salsa
1	head iceberg lettuce, coarsely chopped
1 1/2	cups canned corn, drained

1. In a bowl, combine the fajita seasoning mix, cumin, and salt and pepper to taste. Place the chicken breast in the bowl and turn it to coat it thoroughly. Place the chicken on a microwave-safe plate and microwave it on high for 6 minutes. Remove from the microwave and set aside to cool slightly.

2. In a blender, combine the sour cream and salsa. Pulse until the mixture appears dark pink and has a smooth consistency. (If the dressing is too thick, you may thin it with water.)

3. Cut the chicken breast into 2" pieces. In a large bowl, toss the lettuce, chicken, corn, and salsa dressing together. Serve immediately.

Nutrition Info
Calories: 360
Total Fat: 4 grams
Carbs: 58 grams
Protein: 35 grams
Fiber: 9 grams

Argentinean-Style Steak Salad with Mustard-Cilantro Vinaigrette

Serves 2

Bison steaks are a great lean alternative to beef.

1 1/2 teaspoons Dijon mustard

1/4   cup white wine vinegar

2   tablespoons dried cilantro

6   ounces bison steaks

1   teaspoon each ground cumin and ground coriander

4   bunches watercress

5   radishes, thinly sliced

1. In a small mixing bowl, whisk together the Dijon mustard, vinegar, cilantro, and salt and pepper to taste to make a vinaigrette. Set aside.

2. Season the bison steaks with the cumin, coriander, and additional salt and pepper. Spray a nonstick skillet with cooking spray and place it over medium-high heat. Sear the steaks on each side for 90 seconds, or until a thermometer inserted in the center registers 145°F for medium-rare/160°F for medium/165°F for well-done. (This meat is best served medium-rare.) Remove the steaks from the skillet and let them rest for 1 minute, then slice them.

3. In a large bowl, toss the watercress with the vinaigrette. Arrange the watercress on a plate. Top with the sliced steak and garnish with the radishes.

Nutrition Info

Calories: 433
Total Fat: 7 grams
Carbs: 64 grams
Protein: 35 grams
Fiber: 10 grams

STIR-FRIES

10-Minute Stir-Fry   Serves 2

Simple, satisfying, and infinitely adaptable, this meal should become a staple weekend supper.

TECHNIQUE TIP: Any meat and any veggies will work in this anytime stir-fry.

7	ounces boneless, skinless chicken tenders
2	cups frozen mixed vegetables, thawed
¼	cup reduced-sodium soy sauce
¼	cup reduced-sodium chicken broth
1	tablespoon peanut butter
1	teaspoon cornstarch
1½	cups cooked brown rice

1. Coat a large nonstick skillet with cooking spray and place it over medium-high heat. Stir-fry the chicken for 4 minutes, or until lightly browned but not cooked through. Add the vegetables and stir-fry for 2 more minutes. Stir in the soy sauce.

2. Pour in the broth, then add the peanut butter and sprinkle in the cornstarch. Cook for 2 more minutes, stirring to break up the peanut butter and combine the flavors. Serve over the rice.

Nutrition Info
Calories: 565
Total Fat: 22 grams
Carbs: 65 grams
Protein: 23 grams
Fiber: 5 grams

Creamy Spinach and Chickpea Stir-Fry

Serves 1

This is our easy adaptation of sang paneer, a classic Indian dish. And remember, the spinach will look like a lot when you first put it into the skillet, but it will definitely cook down.

INGREDIENT TIP: Buttermilk lends the creamy texture here—the recipe won't work as well with fat-free milk.

- ½ cup rinsed and drained canned chickpeas
- 2 cloves garlic, minced
- ½ teaspoon ground cumin
- 8 ounces baby spinach, coarsely chopped
- ½ cup reduced-fat buttermilk

  Salt and black pepper
- 2 tablespoons crumbled feta cheese, for garnish

1. Coat a large nonstick skillet with cooking spray and place it over medium-low heat. Cook the chickpeas, garlic, and cumin for 30 seconds, stirring. Add the spinach, cover, and let sit for 30 seconds. Uncover and stir-fry for 2 minutes, or until the spinach is wilted.

2. Stir in the buttermilk and cook until the liquid evaporates. Season to taste with salt and pepper. Remove from the heat and garnish with the feta.

Nutrition Info
Calories: 320
Total Fat: 8 grams
Carbs: 46 grams
Protein: 22 grams
Fiber: 11 grams

Tuscan White Bean and Kale Bruschetta Serves 1

To ensure easy low-fat cooking, invest in a good nonstick skillet. You'll use less oil and need less cleanup time.

SHOPPING TIP: Lots of flatbreads are available in supermarkets— check the Nutrition Facts to compare their fiber contents.

1	cup chopped kale
2	cloves garlic, minced
1/3	cup rinsed and drained canned cannellini beans
1	tablespoon water
1	teaspoon fresh lemon juice
	Salt and black pepper
1	whole wheat flatbread
	Fresh chives, for garnish

1. Coat a medium nonstick skillet with cooking spray and set it over medium heat. Stir-fry the kale for 3 minutes, or until wilted. Add the garlic and stir-fry for 30 more seconds. Add the beans and water, reduce the heat to low, and cook for 1 minute, or until warmed through. Stir in the lemon juice and salt and pepper to taste.

2. Meanwhile, toast the flatbread. Spoon the warm kale mixture over the flatbread. Garnish with the chives.

Nutrition Info
Calories: 310
Total Fat: 6 grams
Carbs: 50 grams
Protein: 22 grams
Fiber: 15 grams

Coconut
Chicken Curry

A quick toasting of the spices brings out the exotic flavors in this super-quick curry dish.

TECHNIQUE TIP: Since everything cooks so quickly, it's a good idea to have all the stir-fry ingredients prepped before starting to cook.

1	tablespoon curry powder
½	teaspoon ground cumin
7	ounces boneless, skinless chicken tenders
1	large apple, unpeeled, cored and cut into chunks
1	cup reduced-sodium chicken broth
½	cup light coconut milk
2	cups cooked barley or brown rice

1. Coat a large nonstick saucepan with cooking spray and place it over medium heat. Stir-fry the curry and cumin for 10 seconds.

2. Add the chicken and apple and stir-fry for 1 minute, or until they are browned and coated with the spices. Add the broth and coconut milk and simmer for 10 minutes, stirring occasionally, or until the chicken is cooked through and the sauce has thickened. Serve over the barley or brown rice.

Nutrition Info
Calories: 400
Total Fat: 7 grams
Carbs: 60 grams
Protein: 27 grams
Fiber: 9 grams

Ginger Shrimp with Swiss Chard and Bell Peppers

Serves 2

Feel free to substitute another leafy green for the chard— spinach, kale, or broccoli rabe are all good options. Note that the cooking time will vary depending on the green used.

SHOPPING TIP: Toasted sesame oil is darker and richer than conventional sesame oil. You need only a small amount for a big flavor boost.

2	teaspoons reduced-sodium soy sauce
2	teaspoons rice wine vinegar
1	teaspoon toasted sesame oil
1	red bell pepper, thinly sliced
8	ounces Swiss chard, trimmed and thinly sliced
2	teaspoons finely chopped peeled fresh ginger
3	tablespoons water
6	ounces frozen cooked shrimp, thawed
1½	cups cooked brown rice

1. In a small bowl, whisk together the soy sauce, vinegar, and sesame oil to make a stir-fry sauce. Set aside.
2. Coat a medium nonstick skillet with cooking spray and place it over medium heat until hot. Stir-fry the pepper for 2 minutes. Add the chard, ginger, and water and stir-fry for 4 more minutes, or until the chard is wilted. Stir in the shrimp and the reserved stir-fry sauce. Stir-fry for 2 more minutes, or until the pepper and chard are crisp-tender and the shrimp is warmed through. Serve over the warm rice.

Nutrition Info
Calories: 355
Total Fat: 8 grams
Carbs: 47 grams
Protein 26 grams
Fiber: 7 grams

Shrimp and Noodle Stir-Fry

Serves 2

*Frozen shrimp is a must-have for quick meals;
not only are the shrimp already shelled and deveined,
they are usually precooked as well. I also like to cook
with high-fiber soba noodles.*

- 2   ounces soba or udon noodles
- ½   red chile pepper, chopped (wear plastic gloves when handling)
- 2   large cloves garlic, minced
- 3   ounces frozen medium shelled and deveined cooked shrimp, thawed
- 1   head baby bok choy or 4 ounces spinach, thinly shredded
- 2   tablespoons frozen green peas, thawed
- 1   tablespoon reduced-sodium soy sauce
- 1   tablespoon sweet chili sauce

1. Cook the noodles according to package directions, then drain.

2. Coat a large nonstick skillet with cooking spray and place it over medium–high heat. Cook the chile pepper and garlic for 1 minute, stirring frequently. Add the shrimp, bok choy, and peas and cook for 3 minutes longer, stirring frequently. Add the cooked noodles, soy sauce, and chili sauce and warm through.

Nutrition Info

Calories: 407
Total Fat: 5 grams
Carbs: 46 grams
Protein: 35 grams
Fiber: 6 grams

Spicy Beef Stir-Fry

Serves 2

*Black bean sauce is a salty-bitter blend of fermented
black beans and garlic.*

½	pound flank steak, cut into 1" cubes
3	tablespoons reduced-sodium soy sauce
3	tablespoons orange juice
2	tablespoons black bean sauce
1	tablespoon sweet chili paste
1	stalk broccoli, thinly sliced and cut into small florets
¼	cup water
4	ounces bean sprouts
1½	cups cooked brown rice

1. In a medium bowl, marinate the beef cubes in 2 tablespoons of the soy sauce for at least 30 minutes.
2. In a small bowl, whisk the remaining 1 tablespoon soy sauce, the orange juice, black bean sauce, and chili paste.
3. Coat a large nonstick skillet with cooking spray and set it over medium-high heat. Cook the broccoli for 2 minutes, stirring frequently. Add the water, cover, and cook for 1 minute, until the broccoli is tender–crisp. Transfer the broccoli to a platter.
4. Lightly coat the same skillet with cooking spray and place it over medium heat. Cook the marinated beef for 2 minutes, stirring constantly. Pour in the black bean sauce mixture. Add the cooked broccoli and the sprouts. Cook for 1 minute, or until warmed through. Serve over the rice and garnish with a sliced scallion.

Nutrition Info

Calories: 470
Total Fat: 16 grams
Carbs: 38 grams
Protein: 45 grams
Fiber: 4 grams

Shrimp and Rice Stir-Fry

Serves 2

If you think Chinese food is unhealthy, think again! This healthy stir-fry beats any takeout.

1	pound shrimp, peeled and deveined
1½	cups cooked brown rice
1½	teaspoons garlic powder
2	cups broccoli florets
¼	cup slivered scallions
2	teaspoons sesame seeds
¼	cup reduced-sodium soy sauce

1. Remove the tails from the shrimp and cut them into bite-sized pieces.

2. Coat a large nonstick skillet with cooking spray and place it over medium-high heat. Cook the shrimp, stirring frequently, for 2 minutes or until cooked three-quarters of the way through. Remove from the heat and set aside.

3. Coat the same skillet with additional cooking spray. Cook the rice and garlic powder for 1 minute, stirring constantly so the rice does not burn. Add the broccoli, continuing to stir. When the broccoli turns bright green, add the shrimp, scallions, sesame seeds, and soy sauce. Cook for 1 minute longer, remove from the heat, and serve.

Nutrition Info
Calories: 407
Fat: 5 grams
Carbs: 44 grams
Protein: 46 grams
Fiber: 6 grams

Endnotes

INTRODUCTION

1 Centers for Disease Control, "42 Percent of Nation to Be Obese by 2030, Study Predicts," CNN Health, May 7, 2012.

2 Lisa Nackers et al., "The association between rate of initial weight loss and long-term success in obesity treatment: Does slow and steady win the race?" *International Journal of Behavioral Medicine* 17, no. 3 (2010): 161–67, doi: 10.1007/s12529-010-9092-y.

CHAPTER 1

1 International Food Information Council (IFIC) Foundation (2012, May 23), "Americans find doing their own taxes simpler than improving diet and health," *ScienceDaily.*

2 Melinda M. Manore, "Dietary supplements for improving body composition and reducing body weight: Where is the evidence?" *International Journal of Sport Nutrition and Exercise Metabolism* (2012).

3 http://news.yahoo.com/body-building-diet-supplements-linked-liver-damage-study-160414178.html.

4 Zerbe, Leah. "Alli weight-loss pills investigated amidst liver damage cases." http://www.rodale.com/alli-liver-damage

5 "10 Diets That Help You Lose Pounds—and Money," *Forbes*, October 10, 2006.

6 Stuart Wolpert, "Dieting Does Not Work, UCLA Researchers Report," *UCLA Newsroom*, April 3, 2007.

7 Eryn Brown, "It's Not Just How Many Calories, but What Kind, Study Finds," *Los Angeles Times*, June 27, 2012.

8 Cara B. Ebbeling et al., "Effects of dietary composition on energy expenditure during weight-loss maintenance," *JAMA*, June 27, 2012, doi: 10.1001/jama.2012.6607.

9 Gary Taubes, *Why We Get Fat* (New York: Anchor Books, 2010), 47.

10 Ibid.

11 John Cloud, "Why Exercise Won't Make You Thin," *Time*, August 9, 2009.

12 James H. O'Keefe et al., "Potential adverse cardiovascular effects from excessive endurance exercise," *Mayo Clinic Proceedings* 87, no. 6 (June 2012), doi: 10.1016/j.mayocp.2012.04.005.

13 Zachary Kerr et al., "Epidemiology of weight training–related injuries presenting to United States emergency departments, 1990 to 2007," *American Journal of Sports Medicine* 38, no. 4 (April 2010): 765–71.

14 T. Finni et al., "Exercise for fitness does not decrease the muscular inactivity time during normal daily life," *Scandinavian Journal of Medicine & Science in Sports* (2012), doi: 10.1111/j.1600-0838.2012.01456.x.

15 Nick Triggle, "Inactivity 'Killing as Many as Smoking,'" BBC News, July 17, 2012.

CHAPTER 2

1 D. J. Jenkins et al., "Effect of nibbling versus gorging on cardiovascular risk factors: Serum uric acid and blood lipids," *Metabolism* 44, no. 4 (April 1995): 549–55.

2 Sonia Gómez-Martínez et al., "Eating habits and total abdominal fat in Spanish adolescents: Influence of physical activity," *Journal of Adolescent Health* 50 (2012): 403.

CHAPTER 3

1 "Superfruits," in *Prevention: The Indian Edition*, May 27, 2008.

2 N. C. Howarth, E. Saltzman, and S. B. Roberts, "Dietary fiber and

weight regulation," *Nutrition Reviews* 59, no. 5 (May 2001): 129–39.

3 "Soluble fiber helps reduce visceral fat. An apple a day, along with a cup of beans, could help reduce the dangerous fat that lies deep in the abdomen and surrounds vital organs," *Duke Medical Health News* 10 (October 17, 2011): 4–5; Christina L. Sherry et al., "Sickness behavior induced by endotoxin can be mitigated by the dietary soluble fiber, pectin, through up-regulation of IL-4 and Th2 polarization," *Brain Behavior and Immunity* (2010), doi: 10.1016/j.bbi.2010.01.015.

4 Christina L. Sherry, Stephanie S. Kim, Ryan N. Dilger, Laura L. Bauer, Morgan L. Moon, Richard I. Tapping, George C. Fahey Jr., Kelly A. Tappenden, Gregory G. Freund. "Sickness Behavior Induced by Endotoxin Can Be Mitigated by the Dietary Soluble Fiber, Pectin, through Up-regulation of IL-4 and Th2 Polarization." *Brain Behavior and Immunity*, 2010; DOI: 10.1016/j.bbi.2010.01.015

5 Marika Lyly et al., "Fibre in beverages can enhance perceived satiety," *European Journal of Nutrition* 48, no. 4 (2009): 251–58, doi: 10.1007/s00394-009-0009-y.

6 J. E. Flood-Obbagy and B. J. Rolls, "The effect of fruit in different forms on energy intake and satiety at a meal," *Appetite* 52, no. 2 (April 2009): 416–22. Epub 2008 December 6.

7 J. Lindström et al., "High-fibre, low-fat diet predicts long-term weight loss and decreased type 2 diabetes risk: The Finnish Diabetes Prevention Study," *Diabetologia* 49, no. 5 (May 2006): 912–20. Epub 2006 March 16.

CHAPTER 5

1 Michael Zemel, "The role of dairy foods in weight management," *Journal of the American College of Nutrition* 24, suppl. no. 6 (December 2005): 537S–46S.

2 D. R. Shahar, "Dairy calcium intake, serum vitamin D, and successful weight loss," *American Journal of Clinical Nutrition* 92, no. 5 (November 2010): 1017–22. Epub 2010 September 1.

3 Carlos Cantó et al., "The NAD precursor nicotinamide riboside enhances oxidative metabolism and protects against high-fat diet-induced obesity," *Cell Metabolism* 15, no. 6 (June 6, 2012), doi: 10.1016/j.cmet.2012.04.022; A. R. Josse et al., "Increased consumption of dairy foods and protein

during diet- and exercise-induced weight loss promotes fat mass loss and lean mass gain in overweight and obese premenopausal women," *Journal of Nutrition* 141, no. 9 (2011): 1626, doi: 10.3945/jn.111.141028.

4 Andrea Josse et al., "Body composition and strength changes in women with milk and resistance exercise," *Medicine and Science in Sport and Exercise* 42, no. 6 (June 2010): 1122–30.

5 Heather J. Leidy et al., "Neural responses to visual food stimuli after a normal vs. higher protein breakfast in breakfast-skipping teens: A pilot fMRI study," *Obesity* (2011), doi: 10.1038/oby.2011.108.

6 University of Illinois College of Agricultural, Consumer and Environmental Sciences (2011, August 11). "Eating protein throughout the day preserves muscle and physical function in dieting postmenopausal women, study suggests," *ScienceDaily*. Retrieved July 25, 2012, from http://www.sciencedaily.com /releases/2011/08/110810153710.htm.

7 D. Paddon-Jones et al., "Protein, weight management, and satiety," *American Journal of Clinical Nutrition* 87, no. 5 (May 2008): 1558S–61S.

8 Alison K. Gosby et al., "Testing protein leverage in lean humans: A randomised controlled experimental study," *PLoS ONE* 6, no. 10 (2011): e25929, doi: 10.1371/journal.pone.0025929.

9 American Academy of Neurology (2011, December 30). "Alzheimer's: Diet patterns may keep brain from shrinking," *ScienceDaily*.

10 http://www.dietsinreview.com/diet_column/08/people-who -maintain-healthy-weights-dont-eat-low-carbohydrates/.

11 N. C. Howarth, E. Saltzman, and S. B. Roberts, "Dietary fiber and weight regulation," *Nutrition Reviews* 59, no. 5 (May 2001): 129–39.

12 Beth Israel Deaconess Medical Center (2012, June 26), "Moderate coffee consumption offers protection against heart failure, study suggests," *ScienceDaily*.

13 Neil Osterwell, "Health Benefits of Coffee," WebMD, August 29, 2011; Youjin Je et al., "A prospective cohort study of coffee consumption and risk of endometrial cancer over a 26-year follow-up," *Cancer Epidemiology, Biomarkers & Prevention* (2011), doi: 10.1158/1055-9965.EPI-11-0766; Fengju Song, Abrar A. Qureshi, and Jiali Han, "Increased caffeine intake is associ-

ated with reduced risk of basal cell carcinoma of the skin," *Cancer Research* 72 (July 1, 2012): 3282–89, doi: 10.1158/00085472.CAN-11-3511.

14 Lap Ho et al., "Dietary supplementation with decaffeinated green coffee improves diet-induced insulin resistance and brain energy metabolism in mice," *Nutritional Neuroscience* (2012), doi:10.1179/1476830511Y.0000000027.

15 Liz Szabo, "Coffee Drinkers May Live Longer, Study Suggests," *USA Today*, May 17, 2012.

16 Jenny Hope, "Junk food fan? Drinking Tea Could Keep the Pounds at Bay," *The Daily Mail*, 20 December 2010

17 Stephen Duffy et al., "Short- and long-term black tea consumption reverses endothelial dysfunction in patients with coronary artery disease," *Circulation* 104 (2001): 151–56, doi: 10.1161/01.CIR.104.2.151.

18 F. Haidari et al., "Effect of green tea extract on body weight, serum glucose and lipid profile in streptozotocin-induced diabetic rats. A dose response study," *Saudi Medicine Journal* 33, no. 2 (February 2012): 128–33.

19 Kimberly A. Grove et al., "(–)-Epigallocatechin-3-gallate inhibits pancreatic lipase and reduces body weight gain in high fat-fed obese mice," *Obesity* (2011), doi: 10.1038/oby.2011.139.

20 L. K. Han et al., "Anti-obesity action of oolong tea," *International Journal of Obesity and Related Metabolic Disoders* 23, no. 1 (January 1999): 98–105; R. R. He et al., "Beneficial effects of oolong tea consumption on diet-induced overweight and obese subjects," *Chinese Journal of Integrative Medicine* 15, no. 1 (February 2009): 34–41. Epub 2009 March.

21 Dietary Guidelines for Americans, 2010. http://www.ers.usda.gov /AmberWaves/November05/Findings/USFoodConsumption.htm; http:// www.ers.usda.gov/Briefing/DietQuality/Availability.htm.

22 Gladys Block, "Foods contributing to energy intake in the US: Data from NHANES III and NHANES 1999–2000," *Journal of Food Composition and Analysis* 17, nos. 3–4 (June–August 2004): 439–47.

CHAPTER 7

1 E. S. Epel et al., "Stress and body shape: Stress-induced cortisol secretion is consistently greater among women with central fat," *Psychosomatic Medicine* 62, no. 5 (September–October 2000): 623–32.

2 R. S. Paffenbarger et al., "Physical activity, all-cause mortality, and longevity of college alumni," *New England Journal of Medicine* 314, no. 10 (March 6, 1986): 605–13; Gretchen Reynolds, "Moderation as Sweet Spot for Exercise," *The New York Times*, June 6, 2012.

3 John Ross, "Forget Pills: Jog Your Way to a Good Night's Sleep," *The Scotsman*, September 17, 2010, 22.

4 Michael Thomas, "Exercise Helps Beat the Blues," *Michigan Chronicle*, November 6, 2010, 6.

5 Dennis Thompson, "To Best Fight Cancer, New Guidelines Urge Exercise; Advice Represents Sea Change from 'Take It Easy' to 'Get Moving,'" *Consumer Health News*, November 5, 2010.

6 T. Heir and G. Eide, "Injury proneness in infantry conscripts undergoing a physical training programme: Smokeless tobacco use, higher age, and low levels of physical fitness are risk factors," *Scandinavian Journal of Medicine & Science in Sports* 7, no. 5 (October 1997): 304–11.

7 G. Finlayson et al., "Low fat loss response after medium-term supervised exercise in obese is associated with exercise-induced increase in food reward," *Journal of Obesity* (2011): pii, 615624. Epub 2010 September 20.

8 K. Ashlee McGuire and Robert Ross, "Incidental physical activity is positively associated with cardiorespiratory fitness," *Medicine & Science in Sports & Exercise* (2011): 1, doi: 10.1249/MSS.0b013e31821e4ff2.

9 American Heart Association, "Overweight, obese women improve quality of life with 10 to 30 minutes of exercise," *ScienceDaily*, March 17, 2008.

10 I. M. Lee et al., "Physical activity and coronary heart disease in women: Is 'no pain, no gain' passé?," *Journal of the American Medical Association* 285, no. 11 (March 21, 2001): 1447–54.

11 "Pedometer Gets People Up and Walking," *The Star-Ledger* (Newark, New Jersey), November 27, 2007.

CHAPTER 9

1 Donna Olmstead, "Give Bones a Boost," *Albuquerque Journal*, August, 9, 2009, 3.

2 F. Mayer et al., "The intensity and effects of strength training in the

elderly," *Deutsches Ärzteblatt International* 108, no. 21 (2011): 359–64, doi: 10.3238/arztebl.2011.0359.

3 R. A. Winett and R. N. Carpinelli, "Potential health-related benefits of resistance training," *Preventative Medicine* 33, no. 5 (November 2001): 503–13.

4 C. J. Mitchell et al., "Resistance exercise load does not determine training-mediated hypertrophic gains in young men," *Journal of Applied Physiology* (2012), doi: 10.1152/japplphysiol.00307.2012.

CHAPTER 10

1 L. Small et al., "A systematic review of the evidence: The effects of portion size manipulation with children and portion education/training interventions on dietary intake with adults," *Worldviews on Evidence-Based Nursing* (June 15, 2012), doi:10.1111/j.1741-6787.2012.00257.x. [Epub ahead of print]

2 M. Murphy et al., "Size of food bowl and scoop affects amount of food owners feed their dogs," *Journal of Animal Physiology and Animal Nutrition* 96, no. 2 (April 2012): 237–41, doi: 10.1111/j.1439-0396.2011.01144.x. Epub 2011 April 19.

3 "Size Can Fool the Eyes: Larger Dishes Can Make It Difficult to Limit Your Portions," *The News-Sentinel* (Fort Wayne, Indiana), November 25, 2008.

4 Nicholas Bakalar, "Servings: Smaller Scoops May Yield Trimmer Waists," *New York Times,* August 1, 2006.

CHAPTER 12

1 A. McTiernan et al., "Self-monitoring and eating-related behaviors are associated with 12-month weight loss among postmenopausal overweight-to-obese women in a dietary weight loss intervention," *Journal of the Academy of Nutrition and Dietetics* (September 2012). Epub 2012 July.

APPENDIX A

1 S. E. Berry et al., "Manipulation of lipid bioaccessibility of almond seeds influences postprandial lipemia in healthy human subjects," *American*

Journal of Clinical Nutrition 88, no. 4 (October 2008): 922–29.

2 S. D. Kunkel et al., "Ursolic acid increases skeletal muscle and brown fat and decreases diet-induced obesity, glucose intolerance and fatty liver disease," *PLoS ONE* (2012), doi: 10.1371/journal.pone.0039332.

3 C. Puel et al., "Prevention of bone loss by phloridzin, an apple polyphenol, in ovariectomized rats under inflammation conditions," *Calcified Tissue International* 77, no. 5 (November 2005): 311–18. Epub 2005 November 16.

4 Nuray Unlu et al., "Carotenoid absorption from salad and salsa by humans is enhanced by the addition of avocado or avocado oil," *Journal of Nutrition* 135, no. 3 (March 1, 2005): 431–36.

5 Rosalie Marion Bliss, "Nutrition and brain function: Food for the aging mind," *Agricultural Research* 55, no. 7 (August 2007).

6 University of Michigan (2009, April 20). "Blueberries May Help Reduce Belly Fat, Diabetes Risk." *ScienceDaily*. Retrieved January 7, 2013, from http://www.sciencedaily.com/releases/2009/04/090419170112.htm

7 Rosalie Marion Bliss, "Researchers study effect of cinnamon compounds on brain cells," USDA Agricultural Research Service, November 9, 2009.

8 Angela Haupt and Kurtis Hiatt, "Greek Yogurt vs. Regular Yogurt: Which Is More Healthful?" *U.S. News & World Report*, September 30, 2011.

Index

Boldface page references indicate illustrations. <u>Underscored</u> references indicate tables or boxed text.

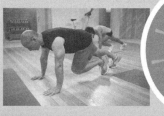
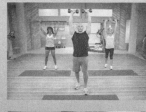
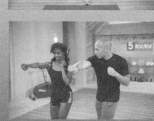
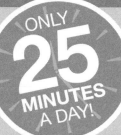
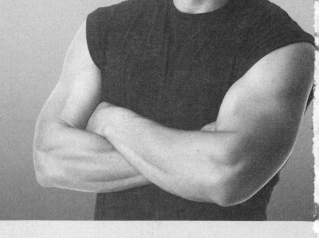